The **Progressive Tinnitus Management** Book

The **Progressive Tinnitus Management** Book

STEP-BY-STEP THROUGH THE FIVE LEVELS OF PTM

James A. Henry

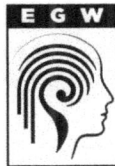

Ears Gone Wrong, LLC

ISBN: 978-1-962629-07-2 (paperback)

ISBN: 978-1-962629-08-9 (ebook)

ISBN: 978-1-962629-06-5 (hardcover)

Contents

Foreword

My professional *"Aha!"* moment came in 2009 as I sat in a Washington DC conference room listening to Dr. James Henry and his fellow researchers present a new method of tinnitus management called Progressive Tinnitus Management (PTM).

The purpose of this meeting was to address the complex issues of traumatic brain injury (TBI), which was commonly experienced by returning Veterans. One of these issues was often the onset of tinnitus. A common scenario is that they would be treated for their TBI symptoms, but the tinnitus remained and became the most prominent issue for them.

Certainly, tinnitus is not unique to Veterans as it also afflicts millions of civilians. As an audiologist in the Veterans Affairs (VA) healthcare system, I was tasked to learn how PTM could benefit our Veterans who had varying complaints about how tinnitus impacted their quality of life. Their complaints included, "I can't sleep," "I can't concentrate," and, on occasion, "I can't live with this any longer—please tell me you can help me." At the time, a common response was, "I'm sorry, there is no cure. You must learn to live with it." I had limited tools to teach them HOW to learn to live with tinnitus. Too often I was left staring into the face of someone who was confused and scared.

I listened intently to Dr. Henry and colleagues describe the principles and protocol of PTM that were based on their years of tinnitus research. I learned about strategies that were available to help people learn how to manage their tinnitus. Education, sound therapy, and cognitive behavioral therapy were all vital components. I also learned the importance of engaging the services of other professionals, which was not commonly done at that time. At that moment I realized I finally had the professional resources and knowledge to help those struggling with tinnitus. I could now confidently say, "I CAN teach you the tools to help you feel better living with tinnitus and improve your quality of life." I could now be a trusted partner in their journey.

As one of the first VA clinics in the country to launch PTM, we spent the early days figuring out how to integrate PTM into our busy clinic. The beauty of PTM is that it is a stepped program to meet individual needs, providing the education and tools to the level at which one needs it. PTM is a stepped-care method, which means one step leads to another and patients only go as far as they need to with the services that are offered. I routinely say, "What works for one person may not necessarily work for another, and PTM is designed to help you discover what works for you, and I can guide you on that path."

I am forever grateful to Dr. Henry and his colleagues, whom I have come to know over the last 15 years. They have provided me with the resources and confidence to successfully help those suffering with tinnitus. I am finding this to be the most impactful and rewarding part of my career.

If you are reading this book as a healthcare professional, someone with tinnitus, or someone seeking knowledge to help a loved one with tinnitus, I am hopeful that you, too, will find your *"Aha!"* moment in the pages ahead.

Cheri R. Ribbe, AuD
Veterans Affairs (VA) Audiologist, Worcester, Mass.

Preface

Fifty years ago, Jack Vernon opened the world's first dedicated tinnitus clinic in Portland, Oregon.[1] At that time less than 10 scientific publications per year focused on tinnitus. Today, a multitude of tinnitus clinics exist around the world, and at least 500 publications per year focus on tinnitus.

In spite of all of this progress over the past 50 years, much remains to be done. Most importantly, we do not yet have a cure for tinnitus. A cure would be some treatment that would eliminate the sound of tinnitus—reliably and safely. The lack of a cure might come as a surprise to people who search the internet for information about tinnitus. Based on an internet search, it would seem that many products are available to "cure" tinnitus. I can only wish that were so.

When visiting a doctor or other healthcare provider, it is expected that competency and expertise are assured by their educational degrees, certification, and licensing. What about clinicians who offer clinical services for tinnitus? Have they received the necessary education about tinnitus management? Are they licensed? Credentialed? Regarding education, the answer is "maybe." Regarding certification and licensing, those umbrella protections do not exist. The reality is that anyone can offer tinnitus services and products, and even claim to be a "tinnitus expert" without any credentials to make such a claim. Buyer beware.

I will acknowledge that there are numerous forms of tinnitus training available for professionals (mostly audiologists). Such training usually involves online courses or in-person seminars. Completing such training ensures a certain degree of knowledge about tinnitus and its management but does not ensure that the clinician is proficient in delivering tinnitus clinical services.

This book describes a method of providing tinnitus services called Progressive Tinnitus Management, or PTM. This method is the culmination of my decades of tinnitus research with contributions from many colleagues.

My first experience with tinnitus was spending six years in the Oregon Health & Science University (OHSU) Tinnitus Clinic, which was directed by Dr. Vernon. This was the "research lab" for my doctoral program between 1988 and 1994. I was already a clinical audiologist, so I had a good understanding of hearing loss. Other than experiencing tinnitus myself, I did not know much about tinnitus prior to this experience.

As part of my doctoral studies I completed two research projects involving testing that an audiologist would do with a patient who has tinnitus.[2,3] Little did I realize at the time that my career was transitioning from being an audiologist to becoming a tinnitus clinical researcher.

I had the good fortune of working at the Veterans Affairs (VA) hospital in Portland, in their auditory research laboratory (later to become the National Center for Rehabilitative Auditory Research). By 1995 I had my first funded grant, and I was now doing tinnitus research full-time. That line of research continued until I retired in the fall of 2022. Since I retired, I have had dedicated time to write books and give presentations about tinnitus.

This book provides education about tinnitus using the specific method of PTM. I have recently written a more general book about tinnitus[4] and a book describing the method of Tinnitus Retraining Therapy (TRT).[5] All three of these books have been written with the rigor that is required for peer-reviewed scientific journals. To make the books easily understandable to all, however, technical and medical terms are minimized—and they are explained when used. The books are thus appropriate for both healthcare professionals and the lay public.

Back to PTM. This book describes PTM in detail. The method involves "steps" of care, with five steps (or *levels*) possible for people with tinnitus.

- **Level 1 Referral**: making sure the person with tinnitus receives the appropriate clinical services
- **Level 2 Audiology Evaluation**: evaluation by an audiologist to assess hearing function and how tinnitus impacts the person's life
- **Level 3 Skills Education**: learning self-care strategies from an audiologist and a psychological health provider to manage the effects of tinnitus whenever it is bothersome

- **Level 4 Interdisciplinary Evaluation**: comprehensive evaluations by both an audiologist and a psychologist to determine why tinnitus continues to be significantly bothersome
- **Level 5 Individualized Support**: one-on-one treatment that can extend the Level 3 counseling or that switches to some other method of treatment

The overall intent of PTM is to provide accurate and efficient assessments of tinnitus and to teach self-help skills to enable individuals to live their lives fully in spite of having tinnitus. PTM has been extensively researched, including controlled trials with over 500 participants (described in appendix A). The method is spelled out in this book, step-by-step. PTM can contribute to the needed standardization of clinical services, credentialing, and licensing to meet the needs of patients with tinnitus. I sincerely hope this book brings clarity about tinnitus and what can be done about it using a method I completely endorse—PTM.

Note to the Reader

This book is intended to provide educational information about tinnitus and related auditory problems. It cannot be construed as providing any form of therapy or treatment. If you have any of the symptoms described in this book and feel that professional services are needed, you should meet with an appropriate healthcare provider.

PART 1

Introduction and Background

CHAPTER 1

Allessia and Dimitri

Allessia works as a dental hygienist. She is in her 40s and has held the same job for about 20 years. About three years ago she noticed her ears were making a sound that she described as "crickets chirping." At first she was not concerned, but the ear noise became more consistent and difficult to ignore. She thought maybe it could have been caused by the tooth-cleaning machine she used with her patients, saying the machine was "not that loud, but it made a very high-pitched sound."

Allessia purchased some yellow foam earplugs, which she put in her ears whenever she used the machine. That relieved her anxiety about the machine making her tinnitus worse. However, she noticed her tinnitus did not let up. She made an appointment with an ear, nose, and throat (ENT) physician who examined her ears. The doctor told her she had sensorineural tinnitus, which is the most common type of tinnitus. Because tinnitus is usually associated with hearing loss, he advised her to make an appointment with an audiologist to evaluate her hearing.

At the audiology appointment she learned that her hearing was normal. The audiologist told her that the ENT doctor's diagnosis of sensorineural tinnitus seemed correct. He added that, in spite of much research, a cure had not yet been discovered for tinnitus. He said that good treatments were available to lessen the effects of tinnitus, such as trouble sleeping and concentrating, and emotional reactions to the intrusive sound. The treatment they offered in their clinic was Progressive Tinnitus Management (PTM), which uses the services of an audiologist and a psychologist. Allessia agreed to sign up for PTM.

PTM is a program that involves five levels (or *steps*) of care. (It is referred to as a *stepped-care program*.[6]) The first level is referral to meet with the appropriate clinician, usually an audiologist. The audiology evaluation is Level 2, which Allessia had already received from the audiologist. She agreed to participate in Level 3, the "skills education" level that meant she would attend a series of five counseling sessions. At this clinic, the sessions were offered in a group setting.

Two of the group meetings were led by the audiologist, who taught the participants how to use sound in specific ways to address different situations when their tinnitus was a problem for them. Allessia thought about the times during the day when her tinnitus bothered her the most. When she was in a quiet environment, the tinnitus seemed to "come out of nowhere." She learned that listening to soothing instrumental music when working at her computer, and nature sounds when falling asleep at night, really seemed to help. She also learned that there are "high-fidelity" earplugs she could use when running her tooth-cleaning machine.

Three additional meetings were led by the psychologist, who provided cognitive behavioral therapy (CBT). (It should be noted that CBT has many different components and only certain ones are offered in PTM Level 3. People who need tinnitus services beyond Level 3 have the option of receiving more comprehensive CBT in PTM Level 5.) In the CBT sessions she learned relaxation techniques, how to engage in activities that would distract her from her tinnitus, and how to think more positively about her tinnitus. She learned this could help reduce her emotional reactions.

She worked to apply what she learned in the classes to her everyday life. During the follow-up phone call with the audiologist, she expressed gratitude for what she had learned. She told him that the meetings were sufficient for her to deal with her tinnitus now on her own, and she wouldn't need any further services at this time.

Dimitri

Dimitri is an automotive mechanic. He has done this type of work all his life, and he is currently 63 years old. He noticed early in his career that he had tinnitus, but he didn't pay much attention to it. He also noticed that he had trouble hearing and went to see an audiologist when he was in his 50s. The audiologist confirmed that he had a "moderate" hearing loss, which explained his hearing difficulties. The audiologist recommended hearing aids, but Dimitri was unable to purchase them at that time.

The audiologist also encouraged him to protect his hearing at work with earplugs. He mistakenly reasoned that earplugs wouldn't help, as he already had hearing loss and probably the damage was done.

Dimitri worked on engines every day. One day, his tinnitus unexpectedly "spiked" in loudness. It stayed at this higher level for the next week, which prompted him to make an appointment with the same audiologist he had seen previously. The audiologist explained that the noise he was exposed to at work was likely the reason his tinnitus had gotten louder. A new evaluation confirmed his hearing had also gotten worse.

The audiologist recommended hearing aids that had a built-in sound generator to address both the hearing loss and the tinnitus—a combination of amplification for the hearing loss and sound therapy for the tinnitus (such hearing aids are referred to as *combination instruments*). Dimitri did not want to wear hearing aids. The whole situation was very discouraging to him—so much so that he decided to retire from his job.

When Dimitri retired, he realized that *his job was his life* and he did not have much interest in anything else. His lack of activity naturally caused him to pay more attention to his tinnitus. He became anxious about it and started having trouble sleeping at night. He started to feel "worn out" from struggling with the tinnitus, and so he decided to visit the audiologist again.

The audiologist explained to Dimitri that she offered Progressive Tinnitus Management (PTM) in her clinic. The audiology evaluation she had done with Dimitri previously was PTM Level 2. She explained that the next step would be to fit the combination instruments that she had recommended before. Dimitri agreed and started wearing the devices. He returned a month later and reported that the sound generator seemed to "take the edge off the tinnitus," but that he still could not stop thinking about it and sleep continued to be a problem.

The audiologist told Dimitri that she could provide tinnitus counseling and that two or three sessions could be helpful. She explained that the sessions would be considered PTM Level 3 *Skills Education*. She also explained that normally a psychologist would provide cognitive behavioral therapy (CBT) at Level 3, but currently no one at the clinic was available to fill that role. Dimitri agreed to the additional help she suggested. She started to provide counseling for sound therapy and was able to teach portions of CBT. She helped explain relaxation techniques and the *planning of pleasant activities*.

Dimitri attended three sessions with the audiologist. He felt that what he learned about sound therapy was helpful, and he made many changes in his life to make sure he was using sound in the best ways to make his tinnitus less of a problem. He especially appreciated learning about *planning pleasant activities*, which motivated him to become involved in a few social activities. He thoroughly enjoyed those and stated that his tinnitus seemed to "fade into the background." All in all, he did much better and told the audiologist he was now able to manage this himself. His life was fulfilling, and his previous distress over his tinnitus had dissipated.

Where Do We Go from Here?

Allessia and Dimitri are two examples from an unlimited number of possible scenarios for people who are seeking professional help for their tinnitus. Each person is unique, and treatment must be adapted to meet individual needs.

> Each person is unique, and treatment must be adapted to meet individual needs.

It should be noted that the information about tinnitus that is found on the internet is often incorrect and misleading. Unfortunately, that's where many people learn about tinnitus when they are searching for answers or to find a tinnitus specialist. They are at a disadvantage if they don't know someone honest and reliable who can point them in the right direction. You might be one of those people. If so, you have plenty of company—the stories are endless of people searching but unable to find the quality help they need. Searching and trying different approaches can be time-consuming and costly.

I have written this book to provide information and resources to people who are struggling with tinnitus. Sometimes what's needed is to just become informed as to how to navigate the "tinnitus terrain."

> information about tinnitus that is found on the internet is often incorrect and misleading

This book is the third in my series under the heading Ears Gone Wrong®. The first is a general book about tinnitus—what it is and what can be done to find relief.[4] The second focuses on a specific form of tinnitus management called Tinnitus Retraining Therapy (TRT).[5] The present book focuses on another form of tinnitus management referred to as Progressive Tinnitus Management (PTM).

Although I am one of the developers of PTM, I cannot claim that it is any more effective than other methods, including TRT, CBT, and Tinnitus Activities Treatment. Nor can I claim that it works any better than counseling from a therapist who is skilled in tinnitus management. What I can claim is that PTM was developed by a team of dedicated tinnitus experts over many years. It was evaluated in major controlled trials (see appendix A), and it has been used extensively within the Veterans Affairs system of hospitals as well as elsewhere. I believe that the information contained in this book can be of great value to anyone who is looking for answers to know how to make tinnitus less of a problem.

> PTM was developed by a team of dedicated tinnitus experts over many years

Suggestions for Getting the Most Benefit from This Book

Although some people may want to read this book from cover to cover, others may get the most benefit by just reading sections that are most applicable to their individual situation. It's important to know, however, that PTM is a stepped-care method, which means one step leads to another and patients only go as far as they need to with the services that are offered.[6]

> PTM is a stepped-care method, which means one step leads to another and patients only go as far as they need to with the services that are offered.

There is great variation between people with tinnitus—how bothered they are and how motivated they are to become informed about their tinnitus. You may just have some general questions about tinnitus, or your life might be turned upside down because of your tinnitus—or anything in between these two extremes. This book should address the entire spectrum of people, who all react differently to their tinnitus. My previous books can answer additional questions.

The Big Picture

I've already alluded to the "big picture" with respect to how people have trouble finding credible information about tinnitus on the internet or anywhere else. Then there is the problem of finding a competent provider who can help them without overcharging them for things they may not need or that have limited or no evidence to justify the cost.

Tinnitus clinical services have come a long way in the past 50 years. They still, however, have a long way to go. The services are anything but standardized, and any clinician can claim to offer tinnitus services regardless of their level of expertise.

How does one find a competent provider? I wish I could point you to a list of verified-competent providers but such a list does not exist. I *can* point you to the American Tinnitus Association (ata.org), which provides free (albeit limited) telephone consultation and also is a wealth of information about tinnitus. That would be a good starting point. Other countries have their own tinnitus organizations. For example, Great Britain has Tinnitus UK (tinnitus.org.uk). Search for these kinds of reputable organizations.

This "Wild West" situation repeatedly points to the need for consumers to become educated about tinnitus. Becoming well informed is your best defense. Be cautious about anything that is said to you or that you might read on the internet. In some cases, bad information is inadvertent due to ignorance. In other cases, people are purposely fraudulent as they attempt to convince you to purchase whatever it is they're selling. This book, and my previous two books, can be used as resources to help you make good decisions to get the help you need for your tinnitus and use your money wisely. It is my sincere hope that this book will help your tinnitus journey be a successful one.

CHAPTER 2

Tinnitus—The Basics

Three questions are asked below as headings in this chapter. It's helpful to have a common understanding of what tinnitus is, how it affects people, and *why* it affects people. I have answered each of these questions in detail in a previous book.[4] In this book I am offering brief summaries in response to each of the following questions.

What is Tinnitus?

The word *tinnitus* is so broadly defined that any type of ear or head noise can be given that label. It needs to be determined whether tinnitus is a *health condition*—meaning a clinical assessment is advised and treatment may be necessary.

For much of my research, we had to determine whether people actually had tinnitus as a health condition. We developed the Tinnitus Screener for this purpose.[7,8] Completing the Tinnitus Screener takes only a minute or two and results in the person being placed in one of five possible categories with respect to ear or head noise. Two of the categories are considered tinnitus—a

> It needs to be determined whether tinnitus is a *health condition*—meaning a clinical assessment is advised and treatment may be necessary.

health condition. The other three categories are considered ear noise—*not* a health condition. The five categories are transient ear noise, temporary ear noise, occasional ear noise, intermittent tinnitus, and constant tinnitus.[4] Each of these categories is explained below.

Transient Ear Noise

Transient ear noise[9] is the perception of a tone that comes on suddenly in one ear, often with a sense of ear fullness and hearing loss. All of these symptoms fade away within a minute or so. This is a completely normal occurrence that is experienced by almost everyone.

Temporary Ear Noise

People often experience *temporary ear noise* after being exposed to loud sound or taking certain drugs.[9,10] Temporary ear noise is usually experienced for up to a week or so and then disappears. It is not a health condition requiring clinical services. If caused by noise exposure, however, it is a warning that damage has been done to the ears and that further exposure could result in permanent tinnitus and hearing loss. Drugs can cause temporary ear noise, but they are usually harmless except for a few *ototoxic* drugs that can cause permanent tinnitus and hearing loss.[11-13]

Occasional Ear Noise

Some people have *occasional ear noise*. This is a gray area that requires a specific definition of tinnitus. My working definition of tinnitus is *ear or head noise that lasts at least five minutes and occurs at least every week*.[4] The main concern is that the ear or head noise lasts long enough to ensure that it is not transient ear noise and that it occurs on a regular basis (at least weekly). If it lasts at least five minutes but does *not* occur weekly, then it is not tinnitus—it is *occasional ear noise*. Occasional ear noise is not a reason to see a healthcare professional.

> tinnitus is *ear or head noise that lasts at least five minutes and occurs at least every week*

Temporary or occasional ear noise should be taken seriously as a potential precursor of tinnitus. If either of these is experienced, the person must be careful to avoid loud sound or to wear ear protection (earplugs and/or earmuffs) when exposed to loud sound—to minimize the possibility that the ear noise will progress to become tinnitus. This is, of course, important advice for anyone to protect their ears from damage.

Constant versus Intermittent Tinnitus

We need to distinguish between tinnitus being *constant* or *intermittent*—the last two of the five categories from the Tinnitus Screener.[7,8]

Some people think their tinnitus is intermittent when it is actually constant. As I've explained in a previous book, "There are at least three possibilities for this discrepancy (and remember, we are talking about *the phantom sound itself*—not about any effects of the tinnitus on sleep, concentration, etc.): (1) The tinnitus is masked (covered up) by sound in the environment. (2) The mind is distracted from thinking about the tinnitus. (3) The tinnitus is more, or less, bothersome."[4] (p. 22)

Primary and Secondary Tinnitus

Next I'd like to address the distinction between *primary* tinnitus and *secondary* tinnitus.[14] So far we've been talking only about primary tinnitus, which we might think of as "dysfunctional nerve activity in the brain that is *not associated with sound waves* and manifests itself as phantom sound."[15] Primary tinnitus is what the great majority of people with tinnitus experience. *Secondary tinnitus* can be thought of as "mechanical activity in the head or neck that *produces sound waves* that are detected by the auditory system via bone conduction."[15] Secondary tinnitus is relatively uncommon[5] and, if it is suspected, requires an examination by an otolaryngologist or other ear-specialist physician because of the possibility of a serious medical condition.[14,16]

How Does Tinnitus Affect People?

People with bothersome tinnitus do not need to be told how it affects them. The reason we ask this question is so clinicians will know how to best target treatment.

Bothersome Tinnitus

Bothersome tinnitus causes people to feel anxious and distressed, affects their quality of life (that is, their ability to function physically, mentally, emotionally, and/or socially), and is enough of a concern to seek some form of help.[4,14]

Tinnitus Questionnaires

At least 10 different questionnaires are used to evaluate how a person is affected by tinnitus.[17,18] Completing any of these questionnaires provides a score—lower scores mean tinnitus is less bothersome, and higher scores mean it's more bothersome.

Creating a tinnitus questionnaire can be challenging because there are so many possible ways that tinnitus can affect a person.[19] The most commonly reported effects are disrupted sleep, emotional reactions, and difficulty concentrating.[4,20]

The various ways that tinnitus can affect a person can be evaluated with relevant questions. Development of the Tinnitus Functional Index (TFI) shows how these different "areas of distress" can be used in a tinnitus questionnaire.[20]

Its development was a major research project involving five test sites and almost 700 patients who completed different versions of the TFI. This four-year effort led to 25 questions that were grouped into eight areas of distress (eight *domains*):

- Sleep disturbance
- Emotional reactions
- Interference with concentration
- Trouble relaxing
- Intrusiveness
- Reduced sense of control
- Hearing difficulties
- Reduced quality of life

Each area of distress receives its own score. Domains with higher scores point out areas of an individual's life that are most affected by tinnitus. That is where treatment should start.

Non-bothersome Tinnitus

Tinnitus is not necessarily bothersome. In fact, about 80% of people who experience tinnitus report it is not particularly bothersome.[14,21,22] We'll discuss *why* tinnitus becomes bothersome for some people but not others in the next section, *"Why* Does Tinnitus Affect People?"

In this book we will refer often to the American Academy of Otolaryngology—Head and Neck Surgery Foundation (AAO-HNSF) because of their key publication in 2014 that recommended clinical practice guidelines for tinnitus.[14] The AAO-HNSF defines *non-bothersome tinnitus* as tinnitus that does not cause anxiety or distress, does not reduce quality of life, and is not enough of a concern to seek help.[4,14] People with non-bothersome tinnitus are typically curious to understand *why* they have tinnitus and *what they might expect* in the future. They mainly just want answers.

It is far too simplistic to think of tinnitus as either being "bothersome" or "non-bothersome."[4] The degree to which a person is bothered by tinnitus can range from "not bothered at all" to "extremely bothered." It is not just one or the other. The "bothered" category is mainly useful to identify people who might benefit from treatment.

> The degree to which a person is bothered by tinnitus can range from "not bothered at all" to "extremely bothered."

Why Does Tinnitus Affect People?

We could ask, "Why does tinnitus affect *some people more than others*?" In short, we're all different and everyone's experience with tinnitus is different. There are many factors that can influence whether people are affected by their tinnitus and, if so, how much they are affected.

> ...we're all different and everyone's experience with tinnitus is different.

What Was Happening When You First Noticed Your Tinnitus?

Tinnitus can start suddenly or come on gradually. If sudden, it might include some significant or even traumatic event. Thinking about the tinnitus may connect the person to the memories of the event. If the event was traumatic, like a car accident, thinking about the tinnitus may trigger all the emotions that followed the accident.[23,24] It's basically the same mechanism that is present in post-traumatic stress disorder (PTSD).[25]

Many people report that their tinnitus appeared suddenly for no known reason, although they might have experienced unusual stress at the time. The feelings of stress that were experienced during the onset of tinnitus might be triggered when thinking about the tinnitus.[26] Even if stress was not a factor when tinnitus was first noticed, the sudden experience of uncontrollable tinnitus can cause anxiety and worry.

Tinnitus that appears gradually is not associated with a single event. Gradual-onset tinnitus often results from long-term exposure to loud sound. The tinnitus might be temporary at first, then become intermittent or constant.[4] At some point it becomes obvious to the person that the tinnitus is not going away. For some, the thought of the sound persisting is a source of great distress. Others know that repeated noise exposure is what caused their tinnitus. They may not give it much thought unless the tinnitus "spikes" in intensity. In general, gradual-onset tinnitus is less bothersome than sudden-onset tinnitus.[27]

How Long Have You Had Tinnitus?

According to the AAO-HNSF, tinnitus that has been experienced for less than six months is considered *recent-onset*.[14] Tinnitus of at least six months' duration is *persistent*. Does it matter whether tinnitus has been experienced for more or less than six months?

It does matter because the longer a person has had tinnitus, the more likely it is to persist. The great majority of clinical trials for tinnitus have required participants to have tinnitus of "at least six months' duration" to be reasonably sure it won't change during treatment. This is why the AAO-HNSF chose six months as the break point between recent-onset and persistent tinnitus.[14]

> ...the longer a person has had tinnitus, the more likely it is to persist

People who are *still bothered by their tinnitus after six months* require special consideration for services because "tinnitus symptoms of 6 months or longer are less likely to improve spontaneously."[14 (p. 13)]

I'll add one more category—*new-onset* tinnitus, meaning tinnitus that has been present for a week or two (and is not temporary ear noise, as described earlier in this chapter).[4] New-onset tinnitus is particularly attention-getting

> People who are still bothered by their tinnitus after six months require special consideration for services...

and can result in focused efforts to understand what's going on and what to do about it.

For someone who experiences new-onset tinnitus, how does that experience change over time? This question relates to the *natural history* of tinnitus, which describes how people typically react to their tinnitus during the months and years following its onset. It is generally understood that most people with new-onset tinnitus will gradually pay less attention to it over time.[28] This means people naturally *habituate* to their tinnitus. Not everyone habituates to their tinnitus, of course, and that's why we're spending time discussing *why* tinnitus affects some people more than others.

What Are Your Personality Traits?

Each person has unique *personality traits*, which relate to how we think, feel, and behave. The topic of personality traits and how they relate to tinnitus is much too complex to address in this short section. I will just say a few words about it here.

Studies have shown that certain personality traits can influence how a person reacts to tinnitus and whether that person is likely to benefit from treatment. In general, people who are prone to being anxious or depressed, or who have sleep difficulties

...people who are prone to being anxious or depressed, or who have sleep difficulties (insomnia), are more likely to be bothered by tinnitus than people without these susceptibilities.

(insomnia), are more likely to be bothered by tinnitus than people without these susceptibilities.[29-32]

What Does Your Tinnitus Sound Like?

Well over 1,000 patients attended the Oregon Health & Science University (OHSU) Tinnitus Clinic in Portland, Oregon. They described their tinnitus most often as "ringing," "hissing," and "clear tone" (www.tinnitusarchive.org). Other common descriptions were "buzzing," "high-tension wire," "hum," "whistle," "ocean roar," and "crickets" or "insects." Many other sounds were mentioned, and in fact, tinnitus can sound like just about any sound in the environment.[4]

Sounds in the environment can be ranked on a scale of "very relaxing" to "very annoying." Typical sounds on the relaxing side of the scale are sounds of nature, such as a waterfall, ocean waves, and chirping birds. Such sounds generally evoke feelings of stress relief and relaxation.[33] Depending on a person's musical preferences, music can make a person feel more relaxed.[34,35] Human voices with certain qualities can have a soothing effect.[36] On the other hand, some sounds, such as squeaky wheels, people arguing, and traffic noise, can induce annoyance and stress.[37]

Do different tinnitus sounds affect people differently? For example, does tinnitus that sounds like a "high-tension wire" cause more distress than tinnitus that sounds like "crickets"? It would certainly seem that some tinnitus sounds would be more annoying than others. There is no way to verify that assertion, however, because people tend to describe what their tinnitus sounds like with respect to how much it bothers them.[4] It's entirely subjective, so we cannot know exactly what a person's tinnitus sounds like, nor can we know if some tinnitus sounds are more bothersome than other tinnitus sounds.

> ...people tend to describe what their tinnitus sounds like with respect to how much it bothers them.

How Do You Spend a Typical Day?

Living a lifestyle that optimizes physical health also improves mental health.[38] Mental health is further affected by stress, relationships, types of activities, and staying busy. In short, the things we think and do in our everyday lives have effects on our physical and mental health.

Some lifestyle factors can easily be controlled or changed through willful effort, while others are more difficult to control or change because of habit or addiction. Regardless, anything we think or do can affect how we react to tinnitus.[39] Some things tend to make tinnitus more bothersome, while others tend to make tinnitus less bothersome. It is therefore important to identify how different lifestyle factors can improve or worsen the tinnitus condition. Let's review some of these factors and think about how they may influence a person's reaction to tinnitus.

> ...anything we think or do can affect how we react to tinnitus.

Are the Sounds You Are Exposed to Helpful or Harmful?

People are exposed to an endless stream of different sounds every day. As a general rule, constant sound can be therapeutic for a person with tinnitus.

Sound therapy is a term that refers to the many ways sound can be used to reduce the effects of tinnitus.[40] The next chapter includes a brief overview of sound therapy and how it is used in one way or another with most forms of treatment for tinnitus. Sound, however, can potentially damage the auditory system. Loud sound is associated with the onset or worsening of hearing loss and/or tinnitus.[41] Music can damage the ears if it is loud enough.[42] Further, just being in a noisy environment can increase stress and elevate blood pressure.[43]

Some people have reactive tinnitus, meaning their tinnitus increases when exposed to sounds that are not loud enough to cause damage to the ears.[4] If this increase in their tinnitus lasts at least until the following day, these people represent a special treatment category with Tinnitus Retraining Therapy.[44-46]

Summary

Tinnitus can be thought of simplistically as the perception of "sound in the ears or head." For many, that's all they know and all they care about. They know the sound is there, and they want it to go away. Making the sound go away would be a cure, which does not yet exist. We therefore have to focus on addressing the effects of tinnitus, which I have referred to many times as being primarily sleep disruption, concentration difficulties, and emotional reactions.

Reducing the effects of tinnitus is the role of treatment. Treatment requires a proper assessment and education so that the affected person is able to make an informed decision about what services might be needed. The education is not simplistic but is essential so that appropriate services are requested and received—no more and no less than what is necessary.

CHAPTER 3

What Can Be Done About Tinnitus?

The list of available treatments for tinnitus is very long. Some treatments claim to eliminate (completely cure) or permanently reduce (partially cure) the *sound* of tinnitus. Such claims are false because no treatment to date has proven to cure tinnitus.[47] We can therefore set these treatments aside and focus on methods that are designed to reduce the functional and emotional effects of tinnitus. These methods can help the person live a normal life in spite of the ongoing tinnitus.

Sound Therapy

In the previous chapter, *sound therapy* was mentioned as referring to the many ways that sound can be used to reduce effects of tinnitus. Some forms of sound therapy are very specific and may involve the use of special devices.

In general, however, just maintaining a background of low-level, non-annoying sound—even while sleeping—is a form of sound therapy. Additionally, hearing aids amplify sound in the environment, which is another form of sound therapy.[1]

Specific methods of sound therapy include *masking*—a method pioneered by Dr. Jack Vernon in the 1970s.[48] Dr. Vernon's original intent was to use wide-band noise (sounds like "shhh") to completely cover up (or mask) the tinnitus. He soon discovered that completely covering the tinnitus was not usually necessary and that *partial masking* (hearing both the tinnitus and the wide-band sound simultaneously) could provide a sense of relief.

> Most methods of tinnitus management use some form of sound therapy as part of their treatment.

Most methods of tinnitus management use some form of sound therapy as part of their treatment.[4] All patients receiving Tinnitus Retraining Therapy (TRT) are advised to avoid silence to reduce the *perceived* loudness of tinnitus and decrease the relative strength of the tinnitus signal.[49] Even the psychological methods of tinnitus treatment generally include the recommendation to add sound to the environment.[50,51]

Notched and Matched Sound

It has been hypothesized that some methods of sound therapy could cause "permanent neural changes resulting in suppression of the tinnitus sensation."[40] [(p. 674)] This bears mentioning because it might be possible to at least partially cure tinnitus using the appropriate stimulation with sound.[4]

One method is to *notch* sound in the frequency region surrounding the pitch of the tinnitus. This has been theorized to reduce hyperactivity in the brain that is thought to underlie the perception of tinnitus.[52] Some studies have notched music in this way.[40] Hearing aids amplify sound, and hearing aids are available that *notch the amplification* around the person's tinnitus pitch.[53,54]

Another method *matches* sound in the frequency region surrounding the pitch of the tinnitus. As with the notching method, the matching method is theorized to reduce tinnitus-related hyperactivity in the brain.[40] Using the matching method, studies have been conducted[55,56] and a commercial product has been made available to use while sleeping.[57-59]

Numerous smartphone apps offer versions of sound therapy.[60,61] The choices are almost endless, with many providing the ability to combine different sounds and listen to guided relaxation. Some offer the notching method.

Established Methods of Treatment

Some methods of treatment have a long history of research and use in a clinical setting. These include cognitive behavioral therapy (CBT and third wave CBT), Tinnitus Retraining Therapy (TRT), Tinnitus Activities Treatment (TAT), and Progressive Tinnitus Management (PTM and Tele-PTM). In my first book in this Ears Gone Wrong® series I have provided a summary of each of these methods as well as my arguments for why I choose to focus on these methods.[4] My second book describes TRT in detail.[5] The present book describes PTM in detail. In the remainder of this chapter I will provide brief descriptions of CBT, TRT, and TAT. I will then discuss bimodal stimulation, which is currently receiving a lot of attention. The remaining chapters will focus on PTM.

If none of these methods is received, can a person still find relief from the effects of tinnitus? Absolutely! I've stated before and will state again that no one method has been proven to be any more effective than any other method.[4,5] Keys to living a normal life in spite of tinnitus are to become informed about all aspects of tinnitus, learn how sound therapy can be helpful for

> ...no one method has been proven to be any more effective than any other method.

you, be skeptical of any product or service that is unproven and/or expensive, and try to meet with a clinician who is knowledgeable and competent in providing tinnitus services and who has your best interest in mind.

Cognitive Behavioral Therapy (CBT)

Treatment with CBT involves a variety of self-help (or coping) techniques. Some of these techniques address the *cognitive* component of CBT and others address the *behavioral* component. The overall purpose of the cognitive component is to identify negative thoughts and beliefs about tinnitus ("thought errors") and replace them with thoughts and beliefs that are more constructive and helpful.[62-64]

The behavioral component of CBT involves engaging in enjoyable activities to shift attention away from the tinnitus and relaxation exercises to reduce stress.[62,64,65] Patients are further educated about tinnitus and hearing loss, how to enrich their sound environment (sound therapy), and how to improve sleep and overall health.[51]

CBT was first introduced as a method to change what people *do* to improve how they feel.[66-68] "Second wave" CBT added the cognitive components to change what people *think* to improve how they feel. Second wave is the traditional form of CBT.[69]

"Third wave" CBT does not attempt to change thoughts and feelings, but rather focuses on becoming more accepting of existing challenges.[66] The objective is not to be relaxed and comfortable but to become disciplined to live in alignment with our beliefs and values even while experiencing discomfort and hardship. Third wave CBT includes mindfulness-based approaches (mindfulness-based stress reduction and acceptance and commitment therapy), which have some evidence of effectiveness in treating tinnitus.[51,70,71]

> "Third wave" CBT does not attempt to change thoughts and feelings, but rather focuses on becoming more accepting of existing challenges.

Tinnitus Retraining Therapy (TRT)

The goals of treatment with TRT are to reduce or eliminate the functional and emotional effects of tinnitus and to become minimally aware of the phantom sound.[46] The word used to refer to these goals is *habituation*—reacting less to the tinnitus and ultimately not being aware of it most of the time.

The TRT evaluation obtains information to place a patient into one of five treatment categories. Selecting the category is based primarily on ranking the degree to which the patient has problems with tinnitus, hearing loss, and decreased sound tolerance.[72]

> *habituation*—reacting less to the tinnitus and ultimately not being aware of it most of the time.

For treatment, TRT uses a program of structured counseling and a specific protocol of sound therapy. The structured counseling is based on the *neurophysiological model of tinnitus*, which underlies everything that is done with TRT and is the most important component of treatment.[46] The model basically explains how different parts of the brain are involved when a person has tinnitus. When tinnitus is bothersome (disrupting sleep and concentration, and causing stress and emotional reactions), some of those brain regions need to be "disconnected." The TRT counseling explains the model in detail.[5,49]

TRT uses a program of structured counseling supplemented with a specific protocol of sound therapy.[5] All patients are instructed to "avoid silence" and to "enrich their sound environment."[5,49] In more severe cases, sound therapy typically involves the use of wearable devices (sound generators) that deliver wide-band noise directly to the ears. The noise is adjusted to a very specific level relative to the tinnitus. Many modern hearing aids have a built-in sound generator, and these are often used for sound therapy with TRT.

Tinnitus Activities Treatment (TAT)

Tinnitus Activities Treatment is described mainly as a specific method of treatment. Various publications also describe how to conduct a tinnitus evaluation for TAT.[73-75] A patient's tinnitus and its history are described in detail using the Tinnitus Intake Questionnaire.[73] Further assessment uses the Tinnitus Primary Functions Questionnaire,[76] which evaluates the impact of tinnitus on thoughts and emotions, concentration, sleep, hearing, and communication.[75,77] A hearing evaluation is conducted along with (if appropriate) a hearing aid assessment. Based on the information from the evaluation, the patient is placed into one of three categories: curious, concerned, or distressed.[73]

The overall focus of treatment is to address the well-being of the patient.[78] Treatment for more severe cases provides counseling specific to tinnitus and its associated problems, along with teaching coping strategies.[73,74,78] Sound therapy, which TAT refers to as *tinnitus partial masking therapy,* is

> The overall focus of treatment is to address the well-being of the patient.

considered optional because of the potential of the added sound to interfere with hearing.[79]

Patients are encouraged to participate in hobbies and activities to distract their attention away from the tinnitus.[75] Some patients use a "tinnitus diary" during the first few weeks of treatment. They are also advised to maintain a background of low-level sound to partially mask the tinnitus and to make it easier to ignore.

Bimodal Stimulation

I have been in this field since the 1980s and am familiar with most of the treatments for tinnitus that have been offered since then. With so many people in need of treatment for tinnitus, it is not surprising that many companies have offered new forms of treatment. The question is always, "Does this new treatment work better than what is already available?"

The latest form of treatment that is currently receiving much attention is *bimodal stimulation*—meaning two modes of stimulation being delivered at the same time. The

> The question is always, "Does this new treatment work better than what is already available?"

basic idea is to deliver a specialized form of sound therapy (acoustic stimulation) along with another mode of stimulation (electrical or tactile/physical) that is purported to enhance the benefit received from the sound therapy. At the time of this writing, two companies are offering a treatment that uses bimodal stimulation. These treatments are fairly new, and I can't predict how they will fare over the coming years. I will therefore make only some general comments without mentioning the companies by name. These comments apply to any new treatments, which are undoubtedly on the horizon.

Placebo Effects

My main concern is whether either of these methods provides benefit that is any better than a placebo. A placebo effect would be benefiting from a treatment simply because the person expected the treatment to work.

Clinical trials that evaluate methods of treatment should ideally be *randomized controlled trials* that include a placebo control group. The placebo treatment should be indistinguishable from the active treatment. For example, if a pill was being tested as a treatment for tinnitus, the placebo treatment would be an identical pill that has no active ingredients. People in the trial would not know if they are taking the real pill or the placebo pill. The current methods of bimodal stimulation have not conducted trials that included a placebo control group. It is therefore not known if these methods work any better than a placebo.

> The current methods of bimodal stimulation have not conducted trials that included a placebo control group.

Controlling Costs

Another concern is cost. Any treatment costs money, but some methods cost much more than others. Moving ahead in steps can be helpful before spending any money on treatment. The first step is to have a hearing evaluation and ideally a medical evaluation from an ENT. These appointments are usually very informative and are often all a person needs to resolve any tinnitus-related concerns. Many people can learn how to self-manage their tinnitus using methods that are either free or very low cost. Other people need some degree of clinical treatment. If these basic approaches are insufficient to resolve a tinnitus problem, then other options can be explored, including the different commercial methods.

> Many people can learn how to self-manage their tinnitus using methods that are either free or very low cost.

Stepped-Care Approach with PTM

A stepped-care approach is used with PTM. Clinical services start with the Level 2 Audiology Evaluation. If treatment is necessary, then Level 3 Skills Education is offered. If further services are needed, then a Level 4 evaluation is done, which determines what treatment should be most helpful during Level 5. Level 5 is the point at which treatment

> Level 5 is the point at which treatment options such as bimodal stimulation would become a consideration.

options such as bimodal stimulation would become a consideration.

Using this stepped-care approach, clinical services are provided only to the degree necessary to meet the needs of the individual. This is an efficient way to go about treatment and can result in significant cost savings. Lower-level services would be the place to start for anyone with tinnitus. Higher-level services would be increasingly tailored to meet the specific needs of the individual.

CHAPTER 4

Overview of Progressive Tinnitus Management (PTM)

PTM is a multidisciplinary and stepped-care program.[6,16] This chapter will describe these basic principles and give an overview of PTM.

Multidisciplinary Care

As already mentioned, it can be challenging to find a clinician who is competent in providing tinnitus services. This is also true for PTM. On the positive side, a survey of audiology doctoral (AuD) programs revealed that 91% of the programs (that responded to the survey) teach PTM to their students.[80] Since 2005, PTM has been described

> PTM is a multidisciplinary and stepped-care program.

in articles, books, videos, brochures, and online training courses.[64,81-83] PTM training seminars have been presented, including at national conferences. It is therefore clear that some audiologists are familiar with PTM. Relatively few psychologists (or other psychological health providers, who are needed at Levels 3, 4, and 5) are trained in PTM.[65]

Audiologists

Audiologists are generally knowledgeable about tinnitus. They can answer patients' questions, and they know what symptoms would indicate the need to refer a patient for a medical evaluation by a physician. Training in the assessment and treatment of tinnitus, however, is not consistent across AuD programs.[84] Fortunately, some AuD programs provide excellent training.[80] Numerous opportunities exist for audiologists to receive tinnitus training at professional conferences, online courses, and focused workshops. Because procedures for tinnitus management are not standardized, the type of training audiologists receive at these venues varies greatly.

As already mentioned, PTM has been described in detail in books, videos, brochures, and an online training course.[64,81,82] My research group and I conducted numerous PTM training seminars around the country. Hundreds of audiologists attended those seminars.

Psychological Health Providers

Psychological health providers (also referred to as mental health providers or behavioral health providers) include psychologists, psychiatrists, social workers, professional counselors, and advanced nurse practitioners. These providers are usually psychologists, and are essential members of the PTM team.[16]

Psychological health providers have two roles in PTM. First, they provide cognitive behavioral therapy (CBT)—a component of the PTM counseling. Some have expertise in third wave CBT, which involves mindfulness-based approaches such as mindfulness-based stress reduction (MBSR) and acceptance and commitment therapy (ACT).[4] Second, they provide diagnostic evaluations of patients who have such severe tinnitus that higher levels of clinical service are needed (only psychologists and psychiatrists are qualified to diagnose psychological/psychiatric conditions).

It is ironic that CBT has the strongest research evidence for treating tinnitus,[62] yet very few psychological health providers have the necessary training and expertise.[85] It would seem logical for audiologists to teach certain components of CBT because they are so commonly the point of contact for people needing help for tinnitus.[62,86] Audiologists could fairly easily learn to teach the *behavioral* strategies of

> It is ironic that CBT has the strongest research evidence for treating tinnitus, yet very few psychological health providers have the necessary training and expertise.

CBT—relaxation and distraction techniques—which require much less training than teaching the *cognitive* strategies (constructively changing thoughts about tinnitus).

Ear-Specialist Physicians

A physical examination by an ear-specialist physician (otolaryngologist, otologist, neurotologist/otoneurologist) is recommended by all clinical practice guidelines for tinnitus that have been published to date.[87-89] The AAO-HNSF stated that the examination "should be directed to identify secondary tinnitus, with potentially treatable or explainable causes, as well as to find signs of serious disease associated with tinnitus."[14] (pS10-11)

Although their recommendation is best practice for ruling out "signs of serious disease," it is often not feasible to send every patient with tinnitus to a physician for a physical examination.[16] Fortunately, as mentioned above, audiologists are trained to know what symptoms would indicate the need to make such a referral. One of the main concerns is the possibility that the patient has secondary tinnitus (see chapter 2).

Stepped Care

Stepped care is a system of delivering clinical services in an efficient manner that ensures that patients receive only the services they need—no more and no less.[6] Some patients require only minimal services. Others require more than that, and they are "stepped up" to receive higher-level services until their needs are met. Stepped-care clinical services create efficiency for both patients and clinicians with respect to conserving everyone's time and resources.

> Stepped care is a system of delivering clinical services in an efficient manner that ensures that patients receive only the services they need— no more and no less.

Clinics that specialize in providing tinnitus services often conduct a comprehensive evaluation with every patient who complains of tinnitus. The evaluation can take hours and may be largely a wasted effort if only minimal services were needed. Stepped care addresses that concern.[6]

Five Levels of PTM

With PTM there are five stepped levels of clinical care, and different providers are involved at the different levels. The five levels will be described in detail in future chapters. This chapter provides a brief overview of each.

Level 1 Referral

Professionals in every healthcare setting (clinics, hospitals, private practice) encounter patients who report the presence of tinnitus. Level 1 applies specifically to healthcare providers and workers who are *not audiologists or*

> Level 1 applies specifically to healthcare providers and workers who are *not audiologists or ear-specialist physicians* (such as otolaryngologists and otologists).

ear-specialist physicians (such as otolaryngologists and otologists).[16,90]

Healthcare professionals who do not have expertise in auditory disorders typically do not know how to respond to questions and concerns expressed by their patients about tinnitus. It is important that these patients are referred to a healthcare provider who has the necessary expertise to address these questions and concerns. Level 1 provides guidelines for referring patients depending on the symptoms reported. Referrals are typically made to audiology, otolaryngology, mental health, and/or emergency care.

Level 2 Audiology Evaluation

The usual starting point for most people seeking clinical services for tinnitus is to meet with an audiologist. All audiologists are highly trained to evaluate and treat hearing loss. As mentioned earlier in this chapter, however, their expertise in evaluating and treating tinnitus varies greatly. This is because training in tinnitus management is not uniform across AuD graduate programs.[84] The PTM Level 2 Audiology Evaluation is a suggested standard for how tinnitus evaluations can be provided in a consistent manner.[91]

The Level 2 evaluation also includes screening for sound-hypersensitivity disorders (most typically *loudness hyperacusis,* which is the inability to tolerate the loudness of sounds that most people can tolerate easily). Sound-hypersensitivity disorders often coexist with tinnitus, and they may require separate services.[92,93]

In summary, the Level 2 evaluation involves only an audiologist who determines whether treatment is needed for hearing loss, tinnitus, and/or sound-hypersensitivity disorders. The audiologist also determines whether the person needs to be referred to another specialty provider.

> ...the Level 2 evaluation involves only an audiologist who determines whether treatment is needed for hearing loss, tinnitus, and/or sound-hypersensitivity disorders.

Level 3 Skills Education

Level 3 provides education about self-managing tinnitus using certain strategies (skills).[82] It is recommended that patients have the opportunity to attend a session of general education about tinnitus prior to committing to the Level 3 program. General tinnitus education is often offered on a regular basis to groups of patients who are considering Level 3 or who may just want to learn more about tinnitus and what options are available for its management. The general education session serves as a bridge between

Level 2 and Level 3 to most efficiently address the needs of patients at this stage of PTM.

Level 3 consists of a series of sessions to teach self-care skills from two different healthcare disciplines.[94] One is from audiologists teaching the use of sound to manage effects of tinnitus.[40] Sound therapy with PTM is unique in that no one particular approach is used.[82] Rather, patients learn how to use sound in a variety of ways to address any situation when tinnitus may be bothersome (*self-directed sound therapy*).

> Level 3 consists of a series of sessions to teach self-care skills from two different healthcare disciplines.

The second discipline is psychology (more generally, behavioral health), which teaches coping skills from cognitive behavioral therapy (CBT).[63] Whereas CBT in general teaches a wide range of different skills, only selected CBT skills are taught in Level 3 (additional CBT skills can be taught in Level 5).[94] Randomized controlled trials that have been conducted to evaluate the efficacy of PTM (see appendix A) have focused specifically on evaluating Level 3.[95,96]

Level 4 Interdisciplinary (Audiology and Psychology) Evaluation

Most patients who complete PTM through Level 3 are satisfied that no additional clinical services are needed for their tinnitus. Some, however, do require further services. If so, they are scheduled to receive a Level 4 Interdisciplinary Evaluation.[82]

At Level 4, patients receive in-depth evaluations to determine why their tinnitus problems persist despite receiving care at Levels 2 and 3. Two appointments are scheduled—one with an audiologist and one with a psychologist. (Whereas any psychological

At Level 4, patients receive in-depth evaluations to determine why their tinnitus problems persist despite receiving care at Levels 2 and 3.

health provider who has expertise in CBT can provide treatment at Levels 3 and 5, psychologists are required at Level 4 because they are certified in diagnosing behavioral health conditions.)

Each evaluation appointment lasts up to about an hour. The audiologist administers the tinnitus questionnaires and a tinnitus-specific interview and discusses the responses in detail with the patient. Further audiology testing may be required. The psychologist administers a battery of tests to evaluate for mental health concerns that may need to be addressed. At the end of each evaluation appointment, the clinician discusses with the patient whether additional treatment is needed and, if so, the patient's preferred course of action.

Level 5 Individualized (One-on-One) Support

Whereas treatment at Level 3 is fairly standardized, Level 5 treatment is open-ended to provide any form of treatment that seems necessary to address the persistent tinnitus

> Level 5 treatment is open-ended to provide any form of treatment that seems necessary to address the persistent tinnitus problems.

problems. One option is to repeat some or all of the Level 3 counseling and take additional time to explain the concepts. The audiologist can go into greater detail about sound therapy and how it might be made more effective in specific situations. The psychological health provider can more fully explain the CBT strategies and/or teach different CBT strategies that were not covered in Level 3.

Another option is to pursue a different form of treatment that seems more appropriate to meet the individual's unique needs. As covered in my previous books, these methods include third wave CBT (acceptance and commitment therapy, and mindfulness-based stress reduction), Tinnitus Retraining Therapy (TRT), and Tinnitus Activities Treatment.[4,5] This would also be an opportunity for the patient to look into other treatment options.

My advice for patients who want to go a completely different direction to receive treatment would be to make a diligent effort to first try any method that is based on research evidence. If none of those methods is successful, then consider other less-evidence-based methods—provided they are relatively low cost and do not have potentially harmful side effects. The last resort would be to go with a commercial product or service that might be costly and more experimental than established methods. The cost, however, should never exceed what can be reasonably afforded, and the person should be fully informed about any potential for harmful side effects.

Summary

PTM is the result of many years of research and experience in the field of tinnitus clinical management. Its genesis was my time spent in the lab and clinic of Jack Vernon and his group in the six years between 1988 and 1994. I was funded in 1995 to conduct independent tinnitus research, and my career since that time focused on tinnitus until I retired in 2022. I was surrounded by colleagues who contributed in countless ways to the PTM protocol. We also had the great benefit of Veterans and other people who gave us feedback and opinions that shaped our thoughts. PTM is thoroughly researched and continually undergoing adjustments to make the program more efficient and effective.

A stepped-care protocol that preceded PTM was first conceived and published in 2005.[83] The protocol was then fully developed, and three books were published in 2010 that described the program in detail.[82,97,98] Some of the methodology draws from Jack Vernon's masking protocol,[48] some from Pawel Jastreboff's TRT program,[49] and some from CBT.[99] Many aspects of the program were developed by me and my research team.

Some guiding principles for PTM are:

1. Stepped care is necessary to address the wide range of how tinnitus affects people.

2. Multidisciplinary care is necessary to address the different components of tinnitus—most generally, audiologists address the auditory components; psychological health providers address the psychological components; otolaryngologists address the medical components.

3. Each level of care is specifically defined except for Level 5 that allows for flexibility in providing different types of treatment. Also, psychologists have flexibility in which measures they use for their portion of the Level 4 Interdisciplinary Evaluation.

4. The overall intent of treatment is to provide education leading to effective self-care.

5. Sound-hypersensitivity disorders (mostly loudness hyperacusis) often coexist with tinnitus and require coordinated management.

The basic treatment protocol for PTM is Level 3 Skills Education.[94] Level 3 has been evaluated in two randomized controlled trials that involved a total of more than 500 participants (see appendix A).[95,96] Both of these trials demonstrated efficacy with the treatment. Level 3 has also been evaluated in clinical settings to determine long-term efficacy with positive findings.[100,101]

PART 2

Evaluation with PTM

CHAPTER 5

PTM Level 1 Referral

A referral is a request to transfer the care of a patient from one clinician or clinic to another. The requesting clinician recognizes that the patient has a health condition requiring the expertise of a different medical specialty.

For our purposes, we need to divide healthcare providers between those who specialize in auditory (ear) disorders and those who do not. We distinguish between auditory and non-auditory healthcare providers because *PTM Level 1 applies specifically to non-auditory healthcare* providers.

The Tinnitus Referral Guide

People seeking clinical services for tinnitus typically meet with an auditory healthcare provider. These include audiologists and ear-specialist physicians such as otolaryngologists, otologists, and neurotologists (see chapter 4).

Some patients, however, report tinnitus to non-auditory healthcare providers. These include chiropractors, dentists, caregivers, nurses, primary care and other physicians, opticians, physical therapists, etc. These non-auditory healthcare providers usually have very limited knowledge about tinnitus. It is not uncommon for a patient to be told by such providers, "Nothing can be done about your tinnitus." To address this concern, the Tinnitus Referral Guide was developed to inform these clinicians (see Table 5-1).

█ **Table 5-1. Tinnitus Referral Guide**

Symptoms:	Refer to?	How soon?
Thoughts of suicide Serious emotional distress	Psychiatrist, psychologist, or emergency care	Immediately, especially if thoughts of suicide
Head injury	Emergency care or ear-specialist physician (otolaryngologist, otologist, neurotologist/otoneurologist)	As soon as possible—ideally within 24 hours
Sudden hearing loss	Audiologist and ENT physician	As soon as possible—ideally within 24 hours ENT treatment may need to start immediately

Symptoms:	Refer to?	How soon?
Symptoms suggest secondary tinnitus ("sound vibrations in the head") Ear pain Drainage from the ear Vertigo	ENT physician	Urgency determined by the referring clinician and ENT physician
Tinnitus plus ALL of the below:	**Should be referred to:**	**How urgent?**
Symptoms suggest primary tinnitus ("nerve activity in the brain"—see chapter 2) No ear pain or drainage No unexplained sudden hearing loss No vertigo No serious emotional problems	Audiologist	Non-urgent Most people with tinnitus also have hearing loss; they should have their hearing tested

This table adapted from the document "Tinnitus: Guidance for DoD Primary Care Providers" developed by the Tinnitus Working Group, consisting of researchers and clinicians from the US Departments of Defense and Veterans Affairs.

The Tinnitus Referral Guide (Table 5-1) is an information sheet that is intended to be used by non-auditory healthcare providers as a quick guide for referring their patients who complain of tinnitus. Using this guide to make referrals should result in appropriate care in most cases. The guide, however, is greatly simplified for use in a busy clinic and is not intended to take the place of clinical judgment.

"Although tinnitus itself is not dangerous, it can be the first sign of potentially dangerous diseases that can even become life-threatening if left undiagnosed and untreated."[102] (p. 382) When a person complains of tinnitus, the relevant questions are, does the person:

- have a serious physical, mental, or emotional condition that requires immediate medical care?
- show symptoms of a non-urgent medical condition that requires a medical examination by a physician?
- show symptoms of a non-urgent psychological condition requiring a mental health evaluation?
- have none of the above symptoms, which would indicate the need for an audiology examination?[82]

Patients may be referred appropriately but may not get the best tinnitus services because there is no official oversight to ensure the quality of these services. It should be noted that clinicians are not required to have any kind of certification to verify their competency in tinnitus management. Even auditory healthcare providers (usually audiologists and otolaryngologists) have different levels of tinnitus expertise and often use very different approaches. Regardless, auditory healthcare providers are at least knowledgeable about tinnitus and can provide any urgently needed services. Ideally, patients referred to these providers would become well informed about tinnitus before agreeing to participate in a program or any medical procedure.[4]

Depending on a patient's symptoms, referral may be made to emergency care, psychological health, otolaryngology, or audiology (or some combination of these). The symptoms may indicate an *emergency* situation (requiring immediate care), an *urgent* condition (requiring care as soon as possible—ideally within 24 hours), or a *non-urgent* condition (requiring care within a reasonable period of time). The following sections address the different symptoms in the order shown in Table 5-1.

> Depending on a patient's symptoms, referral may be made to emergency care, psychological health, otolaryngology, or audiology (or some combination of these).

Psychological Health Referral

Screening for thoughts of suicide (*suicidal ideation*) has become common in primary care and mental health settings.[103] Patients who have these thoughts should be sent to emergency care to receive a psychological evaluation.[102,104]

Many studies have shown that depression and anxiety are common among patients who experience chronic tinnitus.[105-108] These patients may need immediate care. Otherwise, they should be referred to a psychological health provider the same day the symptoms are reported.

Urgent ENT (Ear, Nose, and Throat Physician) Referral

Any person with tinnitus along with symptoms that suggest the possibility of a serious underlying medical condition (see Table 5-1 for specific symptoms) requires an urgent ENT referral.[90]

Head Injury

A blow to the head can cause a variety of different injuries to the auditory structures and/or vestibular (balance) structures.[109] Even a relatively moderate blow can cause permanent hearing loss.[110] A head injury is considered a medical emergency requiring immediate care.[111]

Sudden Hearing Loss

Sudden hearing loss can occur in one or both ears and is often first noticed when waking in the morning.[110,112] It has been reported that tinnitus accompanies sudden hearing loss 91% of the time.[113] The tinnitus may be noticed prior to becoming aware of the hearing loss. If the tinnitus persists, in time it may become more of a concern to the person than the hearing loss.[112]

Sudden hearing loss almost always occurs in one ear and can range from mild to complete loss of hearing.[110] About 50% of the time it is accompanied by dizziness or vertigo (a spinning sensation), which may occur hours or days later. Complete recovery of the person's hearing occurs about 25% of the time, partial recovery 50% of the time, and no recovery 25% of the time. The greatest hearing recovery occurs during the first two weeks.[112] Fortunately, when the hearing recovers it is often accompanied by an improvement in the tinnitus symptoms.

Sudden hearing loss is considered an emergency.[114] It requires prompt diagnosis by an ear-specialist physician (otolaryngologist, otologist, neurotologist/otoneurologist) within one to two days of noticing the hearing loss.[112,115] The physician's office will ensure that an audiogram is obtained the same day to make the diagnosis.[115] Sudden hearing loss can be caused by a tumor, stroke, loud noise, or certain medications. The cause, however, "is often not readily apparent."[112 (p. S22)]

> Sudden hearing loss is considered an emergency.

Treatment of sudden hearing loss, if offered, is also considered urgent.[112,115] Recovery of hearing loss depends on a number of factors, including "time between onset of hearing loss and treatment."[112 (p. S4)] Any delay in treatment can reduce the person's chances of recovering hearing function.[116] Treatment options are numerous and often involve steroid therapy within the first two weeks of symptom onset.[112]

Non-urgent ENT Referral

As mentioned in chapter 3, all clinical practice guidelines for tinnitus recommend that anyone with tinnitus should receive a physical examination by an ENT physician.[87,88] The physical exam is intended to identify secondary tinnitus

and to look for any signs of serious disease.[14] At the very
least, patients with tinnitus need to visit an audiologist.[16]
Audiologists are trained to know what symptoms indicate
the need to be referred for an ENT exam.

Secondary Tinnitus

A primary concern is the possibility of secondary tinnitus.
Unlike primary tinnitus (see chapter 2), secondary tinnitus
is *real* sound that is generated by some abnormality in the
joints, muscles, tendons, or blood vessels in the head or
neck. The sound vibrations are conducted through the skull
and detected by the inner ear (the cochlea).[14]

A "whooshing" sound that pulsates in rhythm with the
heartbeat may be *pulsatile* tinnitus.[90,117] Pulsatile tinnitus can
have numerous causes—one publication listed 26 possible
causes under the categories "arterial," "venous," "temporal
or skull-based," and "other" (including migraine).[117] "A comprehensive evaluation with history, physical exam, and
imaging should be performed in patients with pulsatile tinnitus to rule out important and potentially serious causes
(such as tumors or vascular abnormalities)."[117 (p. 364)] Another
publication listed 20 possible causes of pulsatile tinnitus
and stated, "The diagnostic workup of pulsatile tinnitus is
aimed at ruling out life-threatening abnormalities."[118 (p. 101)]

Some forms of secondary tinnitus are *non-pulsatile*,
which are "much more common than pulsatile tinnitus."[102]
For example, spasming of the tiny muscles behind the eardrum (in the *middle ear*) can cause sounds like clicking,
crackling, buzzing, or even a beating drum.

Another form of non-pulsatile secondary tinnitus can be caused by dysfunction of the Eustachian tube, which links the middle ear to the nose and throat.[90] These tubes normally stay closed, and they open when yawning, chewing, or swallowing—which equalizes air pressure on either side of the eardrum. We typically experience a "popping" noise when the Eustachian tube opens while ascending or descending in an airplane. If the Eustachian tube is the cause of secondary tinnitus, popping or clicking sounds are typically heard along with the sensations of muffled hearing and pressure or fullness in the ear(s). Figure 5-1 shows how the Eustachian tube connects to the middle ear.

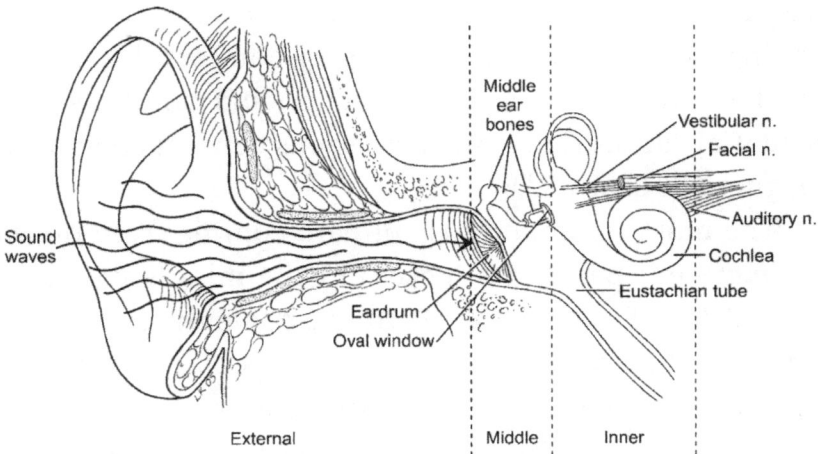

Figure 5-1. Anatomy of the Ear. Sound enters the ear canal and vibrates the eardrum. The vibrations are transmitted to the cochlea via the middle ear bones (hammer, anvil, and stirrup). Hair cells in the cochlea convert the vibrations to neural signals that are sent into the brain via the auditory nerve. The inner ear also contains

| the semicircular canals, which are critical for balance function. (Illustration created by Lynn H. Kitagawa, MFA)

Secondary tinnitus can indicate a serious underlying medical condition that requires the expertise of a physician to diagnose and possibly treat.[14] If secondary tinnitus is suspected, it is essential to receive a medical examination by an ear-specialist physician (ENT/otolaryngologist, otologist, neurotologist/otoneurologist).

Ear Pain

Descriptions of ear pain (otalgia) can range from a deep aching to a sudden and piercing discomfort.[119] The pain can have many causes. "Physicians should rule out several potential causes that can have serious consequences if the diagnosis is delayed."[120 (p. 623)]

The most common cause of pain coming from the ear (*primary* ear pain) is infection of the middle ear (otitis media) (see Fig. 5-1).[120,121] Primary ear pain can also be caused by "swimmer's ear"—which is seen as swelling and redness of the ear canal.[120] Another common cause of primary ear pain is a foreign body in the ear canal such as an insect or small object. Pressure changes in an airplane or while scuba diving can also be a cause.

Potential causes of ear pain due to non-ear conditions (*secondary* ear pain) are numerous. Temporomandibular joint (TMJ) disorder can cause ear pain when talking or chewing.[120] It has been reported that 50% of ear pain cases arise from dental problems.[119] Other potential causes are sore throat and inflammation of the tonsils. Often, the cause of ear pain is unknown.[120]

Drainage from the Ear

Drainage from the ear can be caused by a head injury or by an infection in the external ear or middle ear (Fig. 5-1).[119,122] The appearance of any type of ear drainage indicates the need to be seen by a physician. Infection is the most common cause.[122] Other common causes are runny (liquid) earwax, swimmer's ear, and eczema (dry, itchy, inflamed skin) of the ear canal.[119]

Vertigo

Balance problems can be experienced in different ways. With respect to tinnitus, *vertigo* is the relevant concern.

Vertigo is defined by the sensation of "motion that does not exist."[123] It can be experienced when waking or turning in bed, turning the head while driving, and with certain other head movements. There are many causes of vertigo.[123] One cause that is well known is *Ménière's disease,* which typically has four symptoms that "come and go." They are vertigo, a "roaring" tinnitus, hearing loss, and a sense of pressure in the ears.[110] The onset of vertigo is often sudden and peaks within a few minutes. It may subside within a half hour or last for hours or days (usually two to three hours). It can be triggered by stress, salt, caffeine, and alcohol.[123] It should be noted that vertigo is not dizziness, which is feeling lightheaded.[123]

Referral to an Audiologist

At the bottom of the Tinnitus Referral Guide (Table 5-1) a recommendation is made to refer patients to an audiologist if they complain of tinnitus but do not experience ear pain or drainage, sudden hearing loss, vertigo, or serious emotional distress. The tinnitus should be of the primary type ("nerve activity in the brain") and not of the secondary type ("sound vibrations in the head"). If there is any question, then it is always appropriate to refer the patient to an ear-specialist physician.

If referring a patient to audiology, it is optimal to refer to an audiologist who has expertise in tinnitus management. Although any audiologist can provide basic services for tinnitus, audiologists with special tinnitus expertise will know how to efficiently conduct a tinnitus evaluation during the same appointment. They are also aware of the different options for treatment and can often provide high-quality care on an ongoing basis.

Summary

In summary, I have explained how different healthcare providers can use the Tinnitus Referral Guide (Table 5-1) to know how to refer patients who come to them with symptoms that could be tinnitus-related. I have covered common symptoms that would indicate the possibility of a serious underlying disorder; anyone with those symptoms should visit an ear-specialist physician.[87,88] If a person has tinnitus but none of the symptoms mentioned in this chapter, then the person should at least see an audiologist. The person very likely has hearing loss, which the audiologist can assess. Audiologists are also well versed in identifying symptoms that would suggest the need for referral to an ear-specialist physician.

This completes the description of PTM Level 1 Referral. If a person has tinnitus, then it is appropriate to see an audiologist for an evaluation of tinnitus, hearing loss, and sound hypersensitivity. Such an evaluation is the next step with PTM— that is, the Level 2 Audiology Evaluation. This is the topic of the next chapter.

> If a person has tinnitus, then it is appropriate to see an audiologist for an evaluation of tinnitus, hearing loss, and sound hypersensitivity.

CHAPTER 6

PTM Level 2 Audiology Evaluation

It is reported that up to 90% of people who experience tinnitus are likely to also have some degree of hearing loss.[124-126] For that reason an evaluation by an audiologist is important for any person who experiences intermittent or constant tinnitus (as defined in chapter 2). My research group spent over 25 years evaluating candidates for our research studies, and the PTM Level 2 Audiology Evaluation was developed as a result.[91] Clinical audiologists who have used this protocol have provided feedback as to its efficiency and effectiveness.

> ...up to 90% of people who experience tinnitus are likely to also have some degree of hearing loss.

Overview of PTM Level 2 Audiology Evaluation

The job of the audiologist is to evaluate the patient for three potential concerns: hearing loss, bothersome tinnitus, and sound-hypersensitivity problems.[91]

> The job of the audiologist is to evaluate the patient for three potential concerns: hearing loss, bothersome tinnitus, and sound-hypersensitivity problems.

- If the patient has *hearing loss*, then the audiologist can determine if a hearing aid evaluation is necessary. Hearing aids are the primary form of treatment for significant hearing loss, and audiologists are qualified to dispense them.
- With *tinnitus*, the main concern is to determine whether the person's tinnitus is so bothersome that treatment would be recommended. With PTM, Level 3 Skills Education can be offered.
- *Sound-hypersensitivity problems* can be manifested in different ways as discussed later in this chapter. PTM has methods to evaluate and, in many cases, treat sound-hypersensitivity disorders.

In the process of assessing hearing loss, tinnitus, and sound-hypersensitivity problems, audiologists determine whether a referral is needed to an ear-specialist physician.[90] Even though the published guidelines recommend that a person experiencing tinnitus should receive a physical examination by an ear-specialist physician, audiologists are trained to know what symptoms would indicate the need to make such a referral.[16,87-89] Visiting with an audiologist is usually a good starting point for anyone who experiences tinnitus.

Most basically, the Level 2 evaluation involves a medical history (interview), a short questionnaire (Tinnitus and Hearing Survey), and a routine hearing assessment.[91,127] The information obtained is usually sufficient to know if and how much of a problem the person might have with hearing loss, tinnitus, and sound hypersensitivity. The person may or may not be a candidate for hearing aids. If so, the audiologist can provide them. If the tinnitus is not bothersome, and no referral is needed, then no further services are needed for the tinnitus. If sound hypersensitivity is not a problem, then that potential concern is also ruled out.

> Visiting with an audiologist is usually a good starting point for anyone who experiences tinnitus.

If the tinnitus *is* bothersome, then treatment for the tinnitus may be necessary. The first step prior to treatment is to educate the person about tinnitus, why it can become bothersome, and what treatments are available. Audiologists can provide this information by offering individual or group education and/or educational materials. After receiving this information, if the person desires to go forward with treatment, the options can include PTM Level 3 Skills Education, another method of treatment (see chapter 3), or referral out to a provider who specializes in tinnitus treatment.

This concludes the overview of the PTM Level 2 Audiology Evaluation. What follows in this chapter are details of the evaluation. As mentioned, the basic assessment involves a medical history, the Tinnitus and Hearing Survey, and a hearing evaluation. The assessment may also include the Tinnitus Screener[7] and the Tinnitus Functional Index,[20] both of which are optional as explained further below.

Medical History

The appointment starts with an interview to obtain information from the patient to understand the circumstances and details of any complaints that need to be addressed.

There are no standard questions for obtaining a medical history. Clinicians usually develop their own questions. Personally, I defer to the AAO-HNSF guideline, which includes recommendations for performing a "targeted history."[14] (As a reminder, PTM is eclectic—it draws from many sources, including the AAO-HNSF guideline.) Below is a summary of their recommendations, which I have written about in more detail elsewhere.[5]

Some of the AAO-HNSF's recommendations for conducting a medical history pertain to symptoms of secondary tinnitus (as described in chapters 2 and 5).[14] Such symptoms suggest the *possibility* of a serious medical condition. This possibility either needs to be ruled out or the patient should be medically evaluated by an ear-specialist physician. The following questions can be asked to help rule out the need to refer to an ear-specialist physician.

1. Have you experienced sudden-onset hearing loss (with or without tinnitus)?
2. Is your tinnitus in only one ear or one side of the head (this is called *unilateral tinnitus*)?
3. Do you have unilateral or asymmetric hearing loss (asymmetric being more hearing loss in one ear than the other)?
4. Does your tinnitus sound like it's pulsing along with your heartbeat?
5. Do you experience dizziness or vertigo?

How Long Have You Experienced Tinnitus?

If tinnitus has been present for less than six months, it's called *recent-onset* tinnitus.[14] If it's been present for six months or more, it's called *persistent* tinnitus. Recent-onset tinnitus is more likely than persistent tinnitus to diminish or disappear. Also, the longer a person has had tinnitus, the more likely it is for the effects of tinnitus (such as sleep problems, difficulty concentrating, emotional reactions) to become less of a problem.[14]

Have You Had Significant Exposure to Loud Noise?

Exposure to *excessively* loud noise during work and/or recreational activities can damage the sensitive hair cells in the cochlea, resulting in hearing loss and/or tinnitus.[10,128] Noise exposure can also *worsen* any existing tinnitus and hearing loss. Therefore, it is essential to avoid loud noise or to protect the ears with earplugs and/or earmuffs.

Have You Been Treated with Ototoxic Medications?

Ototoxic refers to drugs/medications that have the potential to damage the inner ear or auditory nervous system. This is mostly a concern with some medications used in hospitals (mostly the *aminoglycoside antibiotics* and the chemotherapy drug *cisplatin*).[12,13] It is known that these drugs can cause permanent hearing loss and tinnitus.[11] Any ear noise triggered by over-the-counter medications is usually temporary. For example, aspirin (salicylates) can cause temporary ear noise but generally only at higher doses.[129]

Have You Felt Anxious or Depressed?

Anxiety and depression can be associated with bothersome tinnitus.[105-108] It is important to determine whether either of these conditions might be present.[14] If they are a potential concern, screening tools are available.[130-134]

Do You Have Trouble Sleeping?

Sleep problems (insomnia) have been reported to be the most common effect of tinnitus.[135,136] The Insomnia Severity Index (ISI) can be used to evaluate the degree to which insomnia is a problem.[137] Addressing sleep problems is essential for many patients, and some need to be referred to a sleep clinic.

Do You Have Trouble Concentrating?

People with tinnitus often complain of concentration diffi-culties.[138-141] More specifically, these are *cognitive* difficulties, which can be measured as performance on a variety of cognitive tests.[139]

Elderly tinnitus patients are at increasing risk for cognitive decline due to dementia. Any cognitive impairment can affect their assessment results and compliance with treatment.[14] It therefore may be important to screen for cognitive impairment using an instrument such as the Mini-Mental State Examination.[142] Suggestions have been made elsewhere for managing cognitive difficulties that are associated with tinnitus.[143]

Does tinnitus *cause* dementia? As just mentioned, the percentage of people with both tinnitus and dementia increases with age. There can be a *correlation* between tinnitus and dementia, but there is no evidence that tinnitus *causes* dementia.

The Tinnitus and Hearing Survey

In each of my first two books in the Ears Gone Wrong® series, I provided a detailed explanation of the Tinnitus and Hearing Survey.[4,5] I always suggest using the Tinnitus and Hearing Survey because it is so effective and efficient in identifying how people perceive their own auditory problems. This one-page survey normally takes only a couple of minutes to complete.

The Tinnitus and Hearing Survey was developed by my research group to address a problem we encountered when recruiting participants for our first clinical trial to evaluate methods of treatment.[144] We needed to determine whether their tinnitus was so bothersome that they would agree to 18 months of treatment to complete the requirements of the trial. We started by screening candidates over the telephone to determine whether they were qualified to come in for an initial evaluation appointment.[144] Screening questions asked them to rate how much their tinnitus bothered them. High scores indicated their tinnitus was a significant problem and treatment was warranted. At the evaluation appointment, we tested their hearing and discovered their main problem was hearing loss. However, they thought the tinnitus was the reason they had trouble hearing, which was not the case.

This scenario of blaming tinnitus for hearing difficulties describes many people today. They have both tinnitus and hearing loss. They are aware of their tinnitus but unaware of any hearing loss. They think their difficulty hearing is because of their tinnitus when in fact it is because of their hearing loss.[145] To address this common problem we developed the Tinnitus and Hearing Survey.[127]

The main purpose of the Tinnitus and Hearing Survey is to determine whether a person has a significant problem with

> The main purpose of the Tinnitus and Hearing Survey is to determine whether a person has a significant problem with tinnitus that is not being blamed on hearing difficulties.

tinnitus that is not being blamed on hearing difficulties.[127] We wrote four statements about tinnitus being a problem that could not be confused with a hearing problem (see Fig. 6-1). Those four statements comprise Section A. They refer to tinnitus interfering with sleeping, relaxing, and concentrating on reading, and the inability to focus the mind away from tinnitus. Note that none of these concerns would be confused with difficulty hearing, so any responses are specific to a tinnitus problem. A score is provided for each item, and the scores are added up. The grand total for the four responses provides a reliable indication of whether the tinnitus *itself* is a significant problem.

Figure 6-1. The Tinnitus and Hearing Survey. Section A determines how much of a problem a person has with tinnitus without blaming the tinnitus for any hearing difficulties.[127] Section B determines whether the person has common hearing difficulties, which would not be conflated with the tinnitus. Section C screens for a sound-hypersensitivity problem.

Tinnitus and Hearing Survey

	No, **not** a problem	Yes, a **small** problem	Yes, a **moderate** problem	Yes, a **big** problem	Yes, a **very big** problem	
A Tinnitus						
Over the last week, tinnitus kept me from sleeping.	0	1	2	3	4	
Over the last week, tinnitus kept me from concentrating on reading.	0	1	2	3	4	
Over the last week, tinnitus kept me from relaxing.	0	1	2	3	4	**Grand Total**
Over the last week, I couldn't get my mind off of my tinnitus.	0	1	2	3	4	
	___	___	___	___	___	
			Total of each column			
B. Hearing						
Over the last week, I couldn't understand what others were saying in noisy or crowded places.	0	1	2	3	4	
Over the last week, I couldn't understand what people were saying on TV or in movies.	0	1	2	3	4	
Over the last week, I couldn't understand people with soft voices.	0	1	2	3	4	**Grand Total**
Over the last week, I couldn't understand what was being said in group conversations.	0	1	2	3	4	
	___	___	___	___	___	
			Total of each column			
C. Sound Tolerance						
Over the last week, sounds were too loud or uncomfortable for me when they seemed normal to others around me.*	0	1	2	3	4	

If you responded 1, 2, 3, or 4 to the statement above:

Please list two examples of sounds that are too loud or uncomfortable for you, but seem normal to others: _____

*If sounds are too loud for you while wearing hearing aids, please tell your audiologist. _____

For office use only (II): ☐ M ☐ H ☐ NS ☐ P ☐ N

This document is available as a free download on the Resources page at https://www.earsgonewrong.org/

The second purpose of the Tinnitus and Hearing Survey is to determine whether the person has significant hearing

> The second purpose of the Tinnitus and Hearing Survey is to determine whether the person has significant hearing problems.

problems. Section B contains four statements that address common difficulties experienced by people with hearing loss—understanding speech when there is background noise, on TV or in movies, in group conversations, and when people have soft voices. As for Section A, the four response scores are added up to provide a grand total for the Hearing section. Comparing totals between Sections A and B provides a realistic picture of how much a person is bothered by tinnitus versus hearing problems.

The third purpose of the Tinnitus and Hearing Survey is to screen for a sound-hypersensitivity problem. The first item in Section C asks if sounds are too loud or uncomfortable when they seem normal to others. If this is at least a "small problem" (that is not due to hearing aids), then the

> The third purpose of the Tinnitus and Hearing Survey is to screen for a sound-hypersensitivity problem.

person is asked to list two examples of these kinds of sounds. An examiner who is knowledgeable about the different sound-hypersensitivity conditions can recommend further assessment if needed.

Audiometric Testing for Hearing Function

Audiometric testing comes after the medical history and the Tinnitus and Hearing Survey. Audiometric testing is routinely done by audiologists to evaluate hearing function and includes testing for air conduction, bone conduction, and speech. To understand the purpose of each of these tests, I'll give a high-level overview of how the hearing system works.

How the Hearing System Works—A Primer

We will discuss the hearing (auditory) system using different analogies to greatly simplify the description of how this extremely complex system functions.[5] Please refer to Figure 5-1 (from the last chapter) for this section.

The ear works like a *microphone* to detect sound in the environment and to convert the sound into nerve impulses that are sent into the brain. Inside the microphone (inner ear, or *cochlea*) is a row of sound-vibration detectors—*hair cells*—spread out like a tiny piano keyboard. Each "key" is a different frequency (or *pitch, tone,* or *note*). For our purposes, we'll imagine that the keyboard represents the entire range of human hearing, with low-frequency tones toward the left and high-frequency tones toward the right.

If a person has *normal hearing*, every key on the keyboard is heard without difficulty. *Complete deafness* would mean that none of the keys are heard no matter how hard they are struck—the keyboard is silent. Normal hearing and complete deafness are the two extremes of the ability to hear. Everything in between would be some degree of *hearing loss*—from slight to profound.

Sticking with our keyboard analogy, hearing loss would involve some keys needing to be struck harder in order to hear them and other keys not working at all. The purpose of the audiometric tests is to determine which keys are not performing properly.

Air Conduction Audiometry

The standard hearing test is air conduction audiometry.[146] This test involves putting an earphone in or over the ears and delivering sound from the earphone to the eardrum. The sound is conducted through the air—hence the term *air conduction*. Each ear is tested separately.

Air conduction evaluates just a portion of the "keyboard." That portion relates to the most critical aspect of hearing—being able to understand what people are saying (*speech*). Speech involves a certain range of hearing, and audiometry generally tests within the range of 250 cycles per second (hertz) to 8,000 hertz.

At each frequency tested, the tone is raised and lowered in a systematic manner to find the softest level at which it can be heard. That level is called the *threshold* of hearing. Thresholds are usually different at different frequencies, and they are plotted on an *audiogram*. With hearing loss, tones have to be made louder (the keys have to be struck harder) before they can be heard relative to someone with normal hearing. Some tones may not be heard at all even when presented at their loudest output level (the keys don't work at all).

Hearing loss is most often seen as high-frequency loss (in the range between 3,000 hertz and 8,000 hertz—toward the right on the keyboard). High-frequency hearing loss would be noticed as difficulty understanding speech in a noisy environment, which is caused by difficulty hearing the consonant sounds ("sh," "th," "s," "f," etc.). Consonants are much softer than vowels ("a," "e," "i," "o," "u") and so they tend to get covered up (masked) by sound in the environment. We must hear the consonants in order to understand speech clearly when there is background sound.

> We must hear the consonants in order to understand speech clearly when there is background sound.

Bone Conduction Audiometry

We normally hear sounds that travel through the air. We can also hear sounds by another route: *bone conduction,* which refers to vibrations (sound waves) in the skull that directly activate the hair cells in the inner ear. Bone-conducted sound bypasses the *middle ear* (eardrum and *ossicles*) that is needed for air-conducted sounds.

We hear our own voice through both air and bone conduction. When we hear our voice recorded it typically sounds "thinner" than what we're used to. That's because bone conduction adds resonance to the sound of our own voice. That resonance is lost when we record our voice.

Bone conduction audiometry uses a *bone vibrator* that's held in position on the bony protrusion behind the ear (the *mastoid bone*).[146] The testing determines whether the middle ear is functioning normally or not. To make this determination, air and bone conduction thresholds are compared. A significant difference between the two (indicating an *air-bone gap*) suggests *conductive hearing loss* (sounds in the air are not conducted properly through the middle ear). If the air and bone conduction thresholds are the same, then there is no air-bone gap and the person has a *sensorineural hearing loss* (typically caused by damaged or missing hair cells). A *mixed hearing loss* would be a combination of conductive and sensorineural hearing loss.

A conductive hearing loss can often be corrected by surgery. A sensorineural hearing loss is generally permanent.

Speech Audiometry

As already mentioned, understanding speech is the most important function of our hearing system. After testing for air and bone conduction thresholds, the next test is speech audiometry, which has two purposes.[146]

First, we want to know the softest level at which speech can be detected—not *understanding* speech but just *detecting* it. This level is called the *speech reception*

...understanding speech is the most important function of our hearing system.

threshold. The test involves listening to spoken words, while wearing earphones, and finding the threshold level at which they can be heard. Below that level they cannot be heard.

Second, testing is done to determine the degree to which spoken words can be understood at a comfortable level. This test measures *speech discrimination* ability (discriminating between different words—also referred to as *speech recognition* ability). To make the test more difficult (and more realistic), background noise can be added to the spoken words to simulate a noisy environment (*speech-in-noise* testing).

Any More Testing?

What has just been described is the minimum amount of testing that is normally required to determine if and what services might be necessary to address hearing loss, tinnitus, and/or sound-hypersensitivity problems.[91] This amount of testing is essentially equivalent to what would be involved with a basic hearing evaluation by an audiologist, plus five or ten minutes to ask questions about tinnitus and to complete the Tinnitus and Hearing Survey.[127]

> Audiologists are qualified to perform a variety of specialized tests to evaluate different components of the auditory system— from the middle ear to the inner ear...

Special Auditory Tests

Many more tests can be performed depending on the results of the basic testing.

Audiologists are qualified to perform a variety of specialized tests to evaluate different components of the auditory system—from the middle ear to the inner ear (shown in Fig. 5-1), and from the auditory nerve to the brain stem, auditory pathways, and auditory cortex. Whole books have been written about each of these tests.

Hearing Aid Assessment

The basic audiometric testing reveals if the person is a potential candidate to benefit from the use of hearing aids. In other words, the hearing thresholds may be poor enough that amplification with hearing aids might improve the ability to hear. If this is suspected, then a *hearing aid assessment* can be performed.[147] Hearing aids can be dispensed if necessary, and more testing is done to ensure optimal performance of the hearing aids.

Testing for Central Auditory Processing

If speech understanding is observed to be worse than what would be expected from the audiogram (showing results from the threshold testing), then it might be suspected that the problem is not so much the damaged or destroyed hair cells, but some problem in the auditory nerve, auditory pathways, and/or the auditory cortex. Special measures are available to test for *central auditory processing disorder.*[148]

Tinnitus Questionnaire

If there is any question whether the person has ear noise that would qualify as tinnitus, the Tinnitus Screener can be used (see chapter 2). The Tinnitus and Hearing Survey[148] does a good job of determining whether tinnitus is bothersome; normally, completing a more lengthy tinnitus questionnaire is not recommended at this stage.[91] Some audiologists, however, routinely administer their favorite tinnitus questionnaires.[18] These are only optional for the evaluation but necessary if the person will be receiving treatment for bothersome tinnitus. (Tinnitus questionnaires will be covered in chapter 7.)

Characterizing the Tinnitus Sound

Many audiologists do testing to characterize the tinnitus sound (referred to as *tinnitus psychoacoustic measures*). These tests include *pitch matching* (identifying the perceived frequency of tinnitus—where is the sound centered on the piano keyboard?), *loudness matching* (matching the loudness of tinnitus to the loudness of an external sound), *minimum masking level* (determining the amount of sound necessary to completely cover, or mask, the tinnitus sensation), and residual inhibition (presenting sound in a certain way to determine whether the tinnitus sensation can be suppressed after the sound is turned off).[149,150] These measures, however, have limited value.[151-154] Mostly, they can be helpful in the counseling process.[151] By "validating" the tinnitus sound with these tests, fears or concerns that are associated with the tinnitus can be lessened.

Testing for a Sound-Hypersensitivity Problem

Finally, completing the Sound Tolerance section of the Tinnitus and Hearing Survey might reveal a sound-hypersensitivity problem.[127] This section *screens* for a sound-hypersensitivity problem. If a real problem is suggested by the patient's responses, then a full sound-hypersensitivity evaluation can be completed using the Sound-Hypersensitivity Interview.[93]

> ...completing the Sound Tolerance section of the Tinnitus and Hearing Survey might reveal a sound-hypersensitivity problem.

Many audiologists perform testing to determine the level of sound that causes discomfort—referred to as *loudness discomfort level* testing.[146] Results of this testing are helpful for determining the maximum output of hearing aids (hearing aids can be adjusted to limit their output to a certain level). Loudness discomfort level testing is also performed with Tinnitus Retraining Therapy and other tinnitus therapy programs.[49,155] It is my recommendation (and that of my research group), however, to not perform loudness discomfort level testing in most instances.[91,93,156] The testing can be very uncomfortable for patients, and results of the testing do not necessarily correlate with real-life discomfort with sound.[157] Real-life problems with sound hypersensitivity can be identified using the Sound-Hypersensitivity Interview.[93]

Making Recommendations Based on the Evaluation

No Treatment Necessary

Treatment may or may not be necessary for hearing loss, tinnitus, or sound-hypersensitivity problems. Ideally, the person (a) will have good enough hearing to not be considered a hearing aid candidate; (b) may have tinnitus but not bothersome enough to require treatment; and (c) will not report a sound-hypersensitivity problem. With these best-case-scenario results, the evaluation has determined that no further services are needed.[91]

> Treatment may or may not be necessary for hearing loss, tinnitus, or sound-hypersensitivity problems.

Hearing Aids

If the person is a hearing aid candidate, then the hearing aid evaluation is performed and hearing aids may be recommended.[147] If the person has bothersome tinnitus, then it would be important to fit hearing aids that have a built-in sound generator.[40] These *combination instruments* do double duty—they provide amplification for hearing loss, and the sound generators can be used to provide relief from tinnitus and to create a constant background of sound to promote *habituation* (consistent with sound therapy used with Tinnitus Retraining Therapy[5,49]). Hearing aids with streaming features are ideal for sound therapy because of the unlimited sounds that are available on the internet.

> Sound therapy can be helpful for both bothersome tinnitus and a sound-hypersensitivity problem.

Treatment for a Sound-Hypersensitivity Problem

If the person has a mild to moderate problem with sound hypersensitivity, then the audiologist would need to differentiate the specific type of sound-hypersensitivity problem (or combination of problems) and recommend appropriate treatment.[93] In most cases some form of sound therapy would help desensitize the auditory system. Sound therapy can be helpful for both bothersome tinnitus and a sound-hypersensitivity problem. If the sound-hypersensitivity problem is severe, then a more intensive treatment program may need to be started.[82,98] A severe sound-hypersensitivity problem should be sufficiently resolved prior to starting specialized treatment for tinnitus.

Treatment for Bothersome Tinnitus

If the tinnitus is so bothersome as to require treatment, then PTM Level 3 Skills Education is recommended.[82,94,98] The next five chapters focus on Level 3.

PART 3

Treatment with PTM

CHAPTER 7

Offering the Option for PTM Level 3 Skills Education

Why Skills Education?

There are many different methods of treatment for tinnitus. I have previously listed methods that are commonly mentioned.[4] That list, however, is far from complete because of the myriad of tinnitus-treatment products and procedures that appear on the internet.

Why *skills education* versus any of these other treatments? To answer this question, we need to first point out that there are two very different approaches to treatment.[158]

One approach to treatment is to ingest some substance or undergo some type of procedure. With this approach, the clinician

...there are two very different approaches to treatment.

provides treatment and the patient *passively receives the treatment*. All the patient has to do is take the pills or show up for clinic visits.

The other approach is to *learn self-care skills,* which means learning how to self-treat the effects of tinnitus. As already mentioned, these effects can involve problems sleeping, difficulty concentrating, and emotional reactions to the persistent sound. The clinician's job is to teach these skills and provide ongoing support as needed. The patient's job is to learn the skills and then apply them as necessary to lessen the effects of tinnitus.

Regardless of whether a person wants to passively receive treatment or to learn and apply self-help skills, the person needs to know that a cure for tinnitus has yet to be discovered.[47] A cure would be complete elimination of the tinnitus sound. Choosing to receive *any* treatment for tinnitus requires an understanding and acknowledgment that *the treatment will not cure the tinnitus* but rather will focus on managing the effects of tinnitus (sleep and concentration difficulties and emotional reactions).

People who are primarily interested in passively receiving treatment are often those who are most intent on being "cured" of their tinnitus. This attitude reflects the popular mindset that doctors should fix any medical problem by prescribing pills or performing surgery or some other procedure. The concept of learning skills and then putting forth the effort to get better may not hold any interest. If this is the mindset, then regardless of how good a treatment is, it will not provide any benefit.

The concept of learning self-help skills is an essential component of educating people about tinnitus and what realistically can be done about it. Before undertaking a program to learn self-help skills, it is essential to provide basic tinnitus education, which can be accomplished one-on-one with the clinician, in a group educational session, or by providing appropriate learning mate-

> The concept of learning self-help skills is an essential component of educating people about tinnitus and what realistically can be done about it.

rial. (My first book in this Ears Gone Wrong® series covers the information I believe people need to become well informed.[4]) Equipped with this information, the person considering PTM Level 3 Skills Education (or any other treatment program) can make an informed decision that will improve the potential for the treatment to be effective.

The Role of Tinnitus Questionnaires

Anyone motivated to be treated for tinnitus by definition has tinnitus that is bothersome enough to warrant treatment. Before anything is done, including being educated about tinnitus (education is a form of treatment), it is important to complete a tinnitus questionnaire. Many such questionnaires have been scientifically validated for measuring how *bothered* a person is by the tinnitus. Tinnitus questionnaires are also used to determine how well a treatment works (its effectiveness).

It should be noted that the Tinnitus Functional Index (TFI) was the first tinnitus questionnaire to be validated for responsiveness[20] (*responsiveness* meaning its demonstrated ability to detect change in how bothered a person is by the tinnitus). Most tinnitus questionnaires are not validated for responsiveness. The TFI is the recommended questionnaire for use with PTM.

If the TFI (or another tinnitus questionnaire) was completed during the Level 2 Audiology Evaluation, then results of that questionnaire can serve as the baseline score against which future scores can be compared. Any reduction in the score would indicate improvement—the greater the reduction, the greater the improvement. It will often be the case that a tinnitus questionnaire completed prior to and following the basic tinnitus education will reveal improvement due solely to the education. The education, therefore, is part of any treatment; education alone may be sufficient to resolve a person's tinnitus concerns.

> ... education alone may be sufficient to resolve a person's tinnitus concerns.

It needs to be emphasized that use of the TFI (or any tinnitus questionnaire) is not sufficient *by itself* for determining the effectiveness of treatment.[159] This is often a point of confusion. It is necessary to pair any reduction in the TFI score with the patient's own impression as to whether there has been improvement.[20] The questions in Figure 7-1 are recommended for this purpose.

We want to se how well our questionnaires captured your true feelings. The questions below will help us understand what you are feeling.

Compared to before I started treatment, my tinnitus now **bothers** me:						
☐	☐	☐	☐	☐	☐	☐
A lot more	Somewhat more	A little more	The same (just as much as before)	A little less	Somewhat less	A lot less

Compared to before I started treatment my **quality of life** is now:						
☐	☐	☐	☐	☐	☐	☐
A lot worse	Somewhat worse	A little worse	The same	A little better	Somewhat etter	A lot better

Figure 7-1. Impression of Change-in-Tinnitus-Impact Questions. These questions are to be asked following treatment for tinnitus. (Adapted from Henry et al., 2024[159])

Summary

To summarize what needs to be done prior to enrolling a patient in PTM Level 3 Skills Education, the person needs to know:

- *There is no cure for tinnitus,* meaning that no treatment can be expected to permanently reduce or eliminate the sound of tinnitus. Treatment therefore focuses on the functional and emotional effects of tinnitus—to get better sleep, improve concentration, and not react emotionally to the phantom sound. The goal is for the tinnitus to have little or no impact on daily life even though the sound is still there.

- *Basic education about tinnitus is essential before deciding whether to enroll in PTM Level 3 Skills Education* (or any tinnitus treatment program). Knowing the facts empowers a person to make an *informed decision* about receiving treatment.
- *Some methods of treatment are known to effectively teach self-help skills.* Treatment involves learning the skills and then applying them in everyday life. Without putting forth the effort, any improvement can only be expected to be minimal at best.
- *A tinnitus questionnaire should be completed prior to the start of treatment.* Treatment would include receiving basic education about tinnitus. Following treatment, the same questionnaire should be completed along with questions about self-perception of change (such as those shown in Fig. 7-1) to determine if and how much improvement has resulted from treatment.

CHAPTER 8

Overview of Level 3 Skills Education

We have now reached the level of PTM that is the actual *treatment* level of tinnitus care. Some people prefer to use the word *intervention* rather than treatment because of the nature of what is done at Level 3. It's called *skills education* because that is what is actually done—people are *taught skills* for how to manage the functional and emotional effects of tinnitus.[82]

All of the previous chapters have led up to PTM Level 3. Clearly, not all patients require the Level 3 intervention. Many, if not most, people who have tinnitus and attend the Level 2

> It's called *skills education* because that is what is actually done—people are *taught skills* for how to manage the functional and emotional effects of tinnitus.

Audiology Evaluation are satisfied that their tinnitus is not enough of a problem to require further services. The next step is to become educated about tinnitus and what can be done about it (which was described in the previous chapter). The education is necessary to make an informed decision whether to pursue Level 3 Skills Education. Basic education about tinnitus is the step between Level 2 and Level 3.

Rationale for Level 3 Skills Education

In the preface and in appendix A I explain the series of events that led to the development of PTM. Some of that historical background is relevant here. In Dr. Vernon's clinic I learned about his masking method of treatment. Audiologists in his clinic completed a comprehensive tinnitus evaluation with every patient. In many cases it was recommended that patients wear "maskers" on their ears that produce a constant level of wide-band noise.[48] The purpose of the maskers was to achieve a sense of relief from any distress caused by the tinnitus. Importantly, their purpose was not to "mask" or cover up the tinnitus, as the name of the method suggests (although covering up the tinnitus was allowable if desired by the patient). Vernon's patients also received fairly extensive, although unstructured, counseling.[160]

A few years after completing my schooling I attended Dr. Jastreboff's training in Tinnitus Retraining Therapy (TRT). The TRT approach is very different from the masking approach. Both methods use sound therapy and counseling, but that's where the similarity ends. With masking, wide-band noise is presented at any level that provides a sense of relief, and counseling is rather unstructured and informal.[125,160] With TRT, wide-band noise is adjusted very specifically to a level that is thought to be best for promoting habituation, and the counseling is very structured and detailed.[5,49] PTM was not developed as a hybrid method combining masking and TRT. Rather, PTM was developed as an entirely new method that offers some components of masking and TRT.[82]

At the time I developed PTM along with my research group, we were aware that cognitive behavioral therapy (CBT) had the stron-gest evidence for treating the effects of tinnitus.[161] It

> PTM was developed as an entirely new method that offers some components of masking and TRT.

therefore seemed obvious that CBT should be included as part of the basic treatment in Level 3. CBT, however, nor-mally requires up to 10 counseling sessions—or even more.[51] For efficiency purposes, we needed to compress CBT down to just a few sessions. Fortunately, CBT consists of a variety of strategies to achieve its objectives. Consulting with a CBT expert, we chose strategies that addressed stress reduction, distraction techniques, and *cognitive restructuring* (thinking more constructively about tinnitus with the goal to reduce its effects).[82,162] These strategies could be taught to patients over three sessions.

We also wanted to include education about sound therapy. The intent was not for patients to use one particular form of sound therapy or to purchase some sound-therapy device. Rather, we felt that patients would be best served if they learned about the different ways sound can be used for treating the effects of tinnitus.[82,94] With that information, they could make a plan for how they would use sound as treatment whenever tinnitus was bothersome. Of course, tinnitus can be a problem in different life situations, and so the optimal use of sound in one situation might not be helpful in another.

We determined that two sessions led by an audiologist would be needed to teach the concepts of sound therapy. During the first session, patients would learn about the various approaches to sound therapy and develop a "sound plan to address their most bothersome situation."[82] They would return about two weeks later to evaluate how well the plan worked, revise the plan as necessary, and potentially develop new plans to address different tinnitus-problem situations.

> People with bothersome tinnitus need to know *what to do* so that the tinnitus doesn't continue to impact their quality of life.

People with bothersome tinnitus need to know *what to do* so that the tinnitus doesn't continue to impact their quality of life. Accordingly, the overall intent of Level 3 Skills Education is to provide patients with the knowledge and skills to know what to do whenever the tinnitus is bothersome.[82] Level 3 accomplishes this for most patients who receive this training.

Overall Structure of Level 3 Skills Education

Each level of PTM was designed to be efficient in addressing individual needs.[82] The Level 2 Audiology Evaluation is straightforward in determining whether treatment is needed for tinnitus, hearing loss (usually with hearing aids), and/or a sound-hypersensitivity disorder.[91]

This chapter makes the assumption that a patient has received the Level 2 evaluation and it was determined that treatment for tinnitus might be necessary. The patient was then educated about tinnitus and the types of treatment that are available. Following the education, the patient and clinician agreed that the patient would benefit by attending PTM Level 3 Skills Education.

Level 3 Skills Education is structured as a series of five sessions for patients to learn different approaches to sound therapy and coping skills from CBT. Two of the sessions are led by an audiologist to teach different approaches to sound therapy and how to create an individualized plan for using sound therapy. Ideally, these two sessions would be separated by about two weeks so that the person has sufficient time to try out the sound therapy plan and then to receive further guidance from the audiologist.

Three of the Level 3 sessions are led by a psychological health provider—usually a psychologist but otherwise any provider who is competent in teaching the principles of CBT. These sessions can be separated by one or two weeks. The five Level 3 sessions are normally scheduled over five consecutive weeks, for example:

- Week 1: audiologist
- Week 2: psychological health provider
- Week 3: audiologist
- Week 4: psychological health provider
- Week 5: psychological health provider

The Tinnitus Functional Index (TFI)[20] is completed by the patient prior to the start of treatment and then again following treatment. Successful treatment would be reflected by a reduction in the TFI score, indicating reduced effects of the tinnitus, which should be verified by the patient's own impression as to whether there has been improvement (Fig. 7-1).[159]

Finally, it is important for patients to evaluate the quality of each session—a form has been developed for that purpose (Fig. 8-1). This form can be used after any counseling or educational session to inform the instructor as to the helpfulness of the session. It's important to provide feedback to the instructors to continually improve the process.

PTM Level 3 Evaluation Form

Please let us know how you feel about today's session so we can meet your health education needs. All responses will be kept confidential and anonymous. Thank you for your time.

Circle your response.

	Strongly Agree	Agree	Neutral	Disagree	Strongly Disagree
1. The instructor was helpful.	0	1	2	3	4
2. The information was useful to me.	0	1	2	3	4

3. I had trouble hearing the information during this session.

Yes   No

4. I had trouble reading the information used in this session.

Yes   No

5. Please share any comments or concerns.

_____

_____

_____

_____

Figure 8-1. PTM Level 3 Skills Education Evaluation Form. This form is intended to be completed by patients and given to the instructor at the end of each Level 3 session.

CHAPTER 9

Level 3 Skills Education: Sound Therapy

Sound therapy is a general term that refers to any use of sound to reduce effects of tinnitus. Effects of tinnitus can vary throughout the day. For example, the tinnitus may seem especially loud and distressing when the person wakes up in the morning. The person may have difficulty concentrating when reading or working at the computer. Or the person may have trouble falling asleep or staying asleep. These and many other everyday life situations can be impacted by tinnitus.

The PTM perspective on sound therapy is that one method of using sound will not be helpful in all life situations impacted by tinnitus. It is not a one-size-fits-all approach. Rather, a specific method of sound therapy is tailored to address each situation when tinnitus is a problem. This approach can be thought of as *situation-specific sound therapy*.

Three Goals for Sound Therapy

Sound therapy with PTM has three distinctly different goals. First, it can provide an *immediate sense of relief* from any reactions to tinnitus. Second, it can *distract the mind* from thinking about the tinnitus. Third, sound therapy can *promote habituation* to become less aware of tinnitus. We will discuss each of these goals and how they are accomplished. Table 9-1 provides a side-by-side comparison of the three goals. As we discuss the goals we will refer to:

> Sound therapy with PTM has three distinctly different goals.

- *Soothing sound* for relief
- *Interesting sound* for distraction
- *Background sound* to promote habituation

Table 9-1. Goals of Sound Therapy for Tinnitus. Although each goal is distinctly different, they typically overlap to some degree. Different sounds can be used at the same time to achieve more than one goal.

	GOAL OF SOUND THERAPY		
	Relief	**Distraction**	**Habituation**
Effects on the person	• Reduced anxiety • Reduced stress • Feel better overall	• Getting the mind off tinnitus and focused on something else	• Reacting less to tinnitus • Being less aware of tinnitus
How can sound accomplish the objective?	If it has a *soothing* effect	If it is *interesting* to listen to and engages the mind	If it is low-level *background* sound that is neither soothing nor interesting
When can the sound be used?	• Any time of day or night • Under any circumstances	• When not performing a task requiring verbal processing (such as reading, writing, etc.)	• Any time of day or night • Under any circumstances
Long-term or short-term effects?	Short-term	Short-term	Long-term

As noted in Table 9-1, using sound to accomplish different goals typically involves some overlap. In other words, a sound used for sound therapy may accomplish more than one

...a sound used for sound therapy may accomplish more than one goal.

goal. The point is to be aware of these different goals and how to accomplish them using sound in different ways. We will now discuss the goals of sound therapy in detail.

1. Relief (Using Soothing Sound)

Soothing sound pretty much describes itself. It is any sound that provides a sense of *relief* from the stress, tension, or anxiety caused by tinnitus. It can also be thought of as *relaxing* sound, whereby just being exposed to the sound evokes a relaxation response. The response would normally be experienced almost immediately upon hearing the sound.

Some typical examples of soothing sound include those that are commonly found in sound therapy apps, such as moving water (waterfall, waves breaking on the shore, babbling brook), nature sounds (crickets, wind blowing through the trees, rainfall), relaxing music, and calming voices used for guided imagery. These kinds of sounds are used for tinnitus relief but are also used for any program designed for stress reduction.

The purpose of soothing sound is the same as for Dr. Vernon's masking method. I explained in chapter 3 how the word "masking" (with respect to sound therapy) is

> The purpose of soothing sound is the same as for Dr. Vernon's masking method.

often misunderstood to refer to sound that covers up (or masks) the tinnitus. Although that was the original intent, Vernon soon realized that sound did not need to cover up the tinnitus to achieve the desired sense of relief. Masking sound = soothing sound = relaxing sound. The masking method has been referred to as *sound-based tinnitus relief.*[163]

2. Distraction (Using Interesting Sound)

As the term indicates, interesting sound is any sound that holds interest to a person. More specifically, it is sound that keeps the person's attention for a reasonable period of time.

The use of interesting sound to reduce effects of tinnitus is a concept borrowed from distraction techniques used for managing chronic pain. "Engaging in thoughts or activities that distract attention from pain is one of the most commonly used and highly endorsed strategies for controlling pain."[164 (p. 90)] Distraction techniques can use different senses including tactile (touch), visual, auditory, or some combination of these.[165] In the case of tinnitus, interesting sound can be a "distractor" that takes the mind off the tinnitus. Not thinking about tinnitus is the practical equivalent to tinnitus being absent.[166,167]

Interesting sound can be used any time it is not necessary to focus attention on reading, writing, or performing any task that requires focused attention involving verbal processing. If the mind is free to wander, it often "locks in" on the tinnitus. Continuing to think about the tinnitus can result in anxiety and stress. It is during these times of emotional distress that

> Not thinking about tinnitus is the practical equivalent to tinnitus being absent.

interesting sound can be helpful to distract the mind away from thinking about the tinnitus.

Because of the stimulating effects, it is often advised to *not* engage the mind when trying to sleep, such as leaving the TV or radio on in the background. Ideally, one would listen to an audiobook that is sufficiently interesting to maintain attention. Podcasts can also be a good choice provided they are not emotionally stimulating. It's a matter of finding speech or other sounds that keep the person's attention without being too stimulating.

3. Habituation (Using Background Sound)

Background sound is any low-level, comfortable, non-annoying sound that is neither "interesting" nor "soothing." It is sound in the environment that does not attract attention and does not provide a sense of relief. Why would such sound be beneficial for dealing with bothersome tinnitus?

The concept of background sound is derived from Tinnitus Retraining Therapy (TRT).[49] I have fully explained the concept elsewhere[5] and will give it a fair amount of attention here. The overall purpose of background sound is to promote habituation of tinnitus. It accomplishes that by contrast reduction, which makes the tinnitus less prominent.

The Concept of Contrast Reduction

We maintain awareness of the world around us primarily by using our eyes and ears. Vision and hearing both operate largely on the principle called *figure-ground perception*. The object being given attention is the *figure*. The figure is placed in a background (the *ground*) of sights or sounds.

As an example, any word that you focus on as you read this page is the figure, and the rest of the page is the (back) ground. The words are written in black ink and the paper is white. Black words on white paper creates maximum contrast to make the words as clear and easy to read as possible.

The example of high contrast from TRT is the "candle in a dark room." If you are sitting in a dark room and there is a candle lit on the table in front of you, the candle flame is prominent because it is so bright compared with the dark background (Fig. 9-1A). The bright candle flame automatically attracts your attention. Now turn on the lights. The brightness of the candle flame has not changed—it's just as bright as before (Fig. 9-1B). The background, however, is now lit up, which *reduces the contrast* between the candle flame and the room. By reducing the contrast, the figure (the candle) becomes less prominent and is consequently less noticeable.

A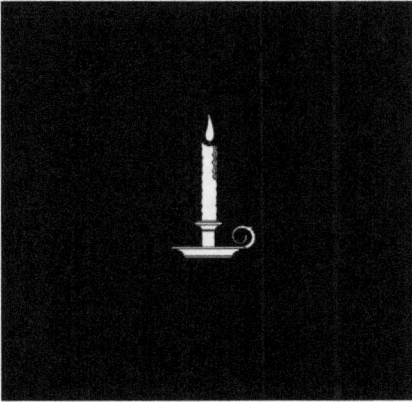

B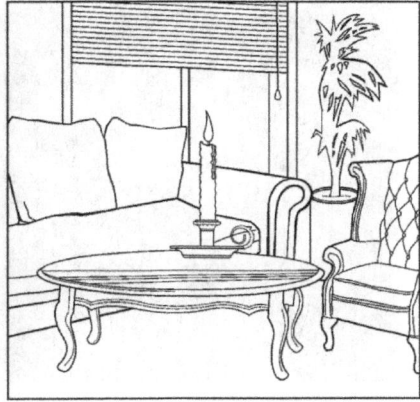

Figure 9-1. Candle Analogy. A. Candle in a dark room (high contrast). **B.** Candle in the same room with the lights on (low contrast). The candle is less noticeable in the lighted room because of the reduced contrast.

Just like the candle can be made less noticeable by turning on the lights, tinnitus can be made less noticeable by adding sound to the environment. Figure 9-2 shows how this works. In the left-hand panel (Fig. 9-2A), the word "tinnitus" is written in white with a black background, which represents quiet. This is a situation of high contrast. In the right-hand panel (Fig. 9-2B), the word "tinnitus" is unchanged but the background is now a light gray. The contrast between the tinnitus and the background has been reduced, which makes the tinnitus less prominent and consequently less noticeable.

> Just like the candle can be made less noticeable by turning on the lights, tinnitus can be made less noticeable by adding sound to the environment.

A
B

TINNITUS

TINNITUS

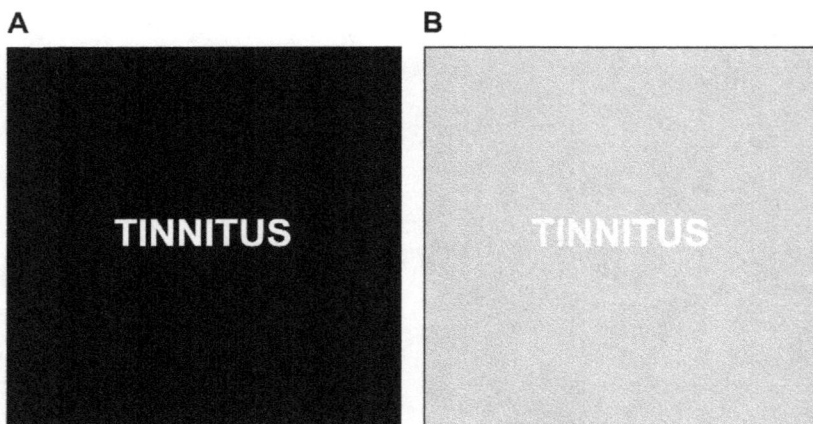

> **Figure 9-2. Tinnitus in Quiet versus in Sound.**
> As for the candle in Figure 9-1, the word "tin-
> nitus" is the same in both panels A and B, but
> it is less noticeable in B because of the reduced
> contrast with the background.

Sound Therapy with Tinnitus Retraining Therapy

Sound therapy with TRT is done in a very specific manner.[5,49] Patients are advised to "avoid silence" and to be exposed to background sound 24/7. The proper use of sound combined with the structured and detailed counseling is designed to promote *habituation*—the stated goal of TRT. We naturally habituate to sounds that are essentially meaningless with respect to our everyday activities. Those kinds of sounds are there in the background, but we normally do not pay attention to them. The idea with TRT is to retrain the brain to "classify" (respond to) tinnitus in the same way as for any meaningless sound.

Another important concept from TRT is that *sound therapy should not change the sound of the tinnitus*. This

concept is often misun-
derstood, so I'm going to
explain it in some detail.
We've discussed the method
of *masking*, which was pioneered by Jack Vernon. His
approach was to use sound
(usually wide-band noise

> The idea with TRT is to retrain the brain to "classify" (respond to) tinnitus in the same way as for any meaningless sound.

from ear-level "maskers") to provide a sense of relief from
any emotional reactions caused by the tinnitus. With TRT
the word *suppression* is used rather than masking to be more
accurate with respect to the effect of sound on the neural
activity underlying tinnitus.[46,168]

With respect to suppression of tinnitus, sound can cause
one of three effects: *complete suppression* (tinnitus cannot be
heard—it's covered up by the sound), *partial suppression* (the
sound and the tinnitus mix together such that *the tinnitus
sounds different*), or *no suppression* (the tinnitus sensation
does not change) (Fig. 9-3). Any external sound that is perceived by the person with tinnitus can be placed into one of
these three categories. What is often difficult for people is
knowing *when* "the tinnitus sounds different."

Louder

Complete Suppression
Complete elimination of tinnitus
perception

Inappropriate
range for TRT

Partial Suppression
Spectral changes in tinnitus sound -
with or without reduced perception
of tinnitus loudness

(not to scale)

Mixing range -
inappropriate
for TRT

◄ **Mixing Point**

No Suppression
No spectral changes in tinnitus
sound - with or without reduced
perception of tinnitus loudness

**Appropriate
range for TRT**

Softer

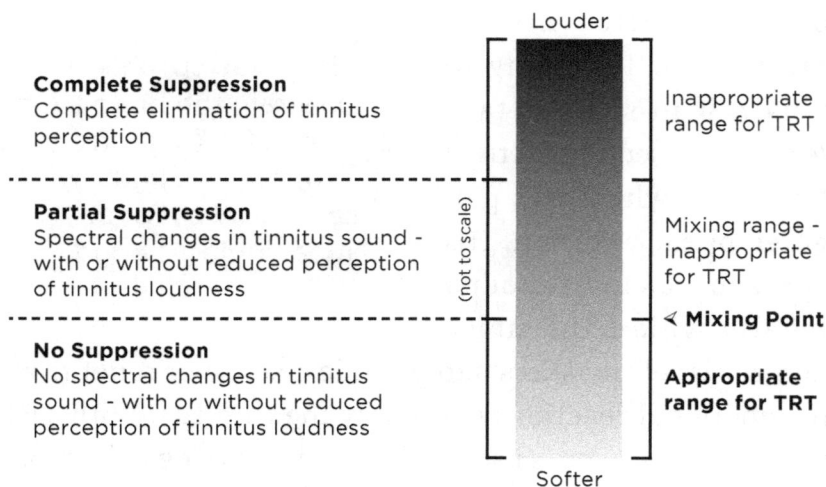

Figure 9-3. Effects of Sound on Suppressing Tinnitus. As sound is made louder, there are three ranges with respect to how sound affects the tinnitus sensation. (Note that any change in the perceived *loudness* of the tinnitus is irrelevant.) In the "no-suppression" range the sound does not change what the tinnitus sounds like. As the sound is made louder, at some point (the "mixing point") the sound of the tinnitus starts to change. Above the mixing point is the "partial-suppression" range. As the sound is made louder, "complete suppression" of tinnitus occurs (for most people). In this highest range, the tinnitus cannot be heard at all. For sound therapy with TRT, sound must be below the mixing point (in the no-suppression range) to promote habituation to the usual tinnitus sound. (Illustration created by Lynn H. Kitagawa, MFA)

Tinnitus sounding different does *not* mean that the perceived loudness of the tinnitus has changed. What it *does* mean is that its quality or *timbre* has changed. Imagine you have sound generators on your ears and switch one of them on. At first you don't hear anything. As you slowly turn up the volume, you begin to hear the wide-band noise. It is very soft, and the noise and your tinnitus sound distinctly different. As you continue to turn up the volume, at some point the noise and your tinnitus start to mix, or blend, together—the noise *distorts or interferes with* the tinnitus.[169] That is the point at which the sound of the tinnitus starts to change, which, according to TRT, is the *mixing point*. What's important about the mixing point?

To answer that question, let's go to the source (Jastreboff and Hazell's TRT book): "It is important to preserve the original tinnitus signal. When the tinnitus signal is modified, even if it is habituated, once the external sound source is removed, the tinnitus will return to its original unhabituated state. Consequently, there will be only a partial decrease of reaction to tinnitus, based on the generalization principle. In the extreme case when the tinnitus signal is totally suppressed, by definition habituation cannot occur. When the sound level does not totally suppress the tinnitus but partly alters it, so-called 'partial masking' (Moore 1995), habituation may occur, but its effectiveness is decreased and less predictable, as the signal to be habituated will be different from the original one."[49] (pp. 116-117)

This is how I might rephrase what Drs. Jastreboff and Hazell are saying: To optimize habituation to the tinnitus, the tinnitus sound needs to remain unchanged from what it normally sounds like. If the tinnitus sound is changed (in the partial-suppression range above the mixing point) during sound therapy, then habituation may wrongly occur *to the modified tinnitus sound.* When removing the external sound, the tinnitus goes back to sounding like it normally does (its usual sound). Although some habituation may have taken place to the *modified* tinnitus sound, it has not taken place to the *usual* tinnitus sound. Furthermore, using sound to completely suppress tinnitus means that habituation cannot occur at all. In summary:

- **Complete suppression** of tinnitus would result in no habituation.
- **Partial suppression** would result in habituation of the modified tinnitus but not of the usual tinnitus.
- **No suppression** would result in habituation of the usual sound of the tinnitus, which is the objective of TRT.

The argument from TRT that sound therapy must occur below the mixing point to promote habituation is based on scientific reasoning. To date, however, it is a theory that has not been proven. With PTM, patients should understand how sound therapy is used with TRT. They need to be informed about that approach, and then they can either try diligently to have 24/7 exposure to sound that is always below the mixing point or just use background sound in general without attempting to achieve the precise level that is used with TRT. It generally takes practice to identify the mixing point and to know if the sound used for therapy is above or below the mixing point.

One additional point from TRT is that ear-level sound generators (or hearing aids with built-in sound generators) are considered ideal for sound therapy because the sound output from the devices can be adjusted to be just under the mixing point. Although sound in the environment might change, the sound level from the sound generators remains constant throughout the day.

Soothing, Interesting, and Background Sounds Often Overlap

As mentioned earlier in this chapter, using sound can accomplish more than one goal (Table 9-1). Whether this occurs depends on the purpose for the particular sound chosen. Soothing sound can make a person feel better and also serve as background sound. Interesting sound can keep a person's attention and also serve as background sound. Background sound, however, is neither soothing nor interesting.

It's also possible to use background sound continually but to add soothing or interesting sound as needed. By maintaining constant background sound, the tinnitus is made less noticeable, which is due to the decreased contrast between the tinnitus and the surrounding sound environment (Fig. 9-2).

Three Sources of Sound

I have described three approaches to using sound as therapy: soothing sound to achieve an immediate sense of relief, interesting sound to distract the mind from tinnitus, and background sound to promote habituation. We will now expand on this framework to describe how different *sources*

> There are three general sources of sound: environmental, music, and voices.

of sounds can be used for each of these approaches. There are three general sources of sound: environmental, music, and voices. I will explain each of these sources and provide examples. The main point here is that sounds in each of these sources can be used to accomplish the goals of relief, distraction, and habituation. We can envision a three-by-three grid, which shows nine combinations of sounds that can be used as sound therapy for tinnitus. We refer to this as the *sound grid* (Table 9-2).

Table 9-2. The Sound Grid. Three *goals* for using sound (*relief* with soothing sound, *distraction* with interesting sound, *habituation* with background sound) can be used to manage reactions to tinnitus. Each goal can use sounds from the *sources* of *environmental* sound, *music*, and/or *voices* depending on what combination works best for a particular tinnitus-problem situation. The checkmarks show that a total of nine combinations of goals for using sound and sources of sound are possible for use as sound therapy.

	Source of Sound		
Goal of Sound Therapy	Environ- mental	Music	Voices
Relief (using soothing sound)	✓	✓	✓
Distraction (using interesting sound)	✓	✓	✓
Habituation (using background sound)	✓	✓	✓

Environmental sound, music, and voices are mostly self-explanatory. Environmental sound is distinguished by not being musical and not created by the human voice. It can be either sounds of nature or synthetic sounds. Sounds of nature would include animal sounds, weather, moving water, etc. Synthetic sounds are those generated by devices made by humans, such as masking noise, wind chimes, fan noise, traffic noise, radio static, or a bubbling fish tank. Environmental sound can be used as soothing sound, interesting sound, and/or background sound. Examples of each are shown in Table 9-3.

Table 9-3. Examples of Sounds in the Sound Grid. Everyone's preferences and reactions to sounds are highly individualized. The examples are only suggestions to assist in discovering sounds that might be helpful to you. The examples shown fit into the nine different combinations shown in the sound grid (Table 9-2).

Goal of Sound Therapy	Source of Sound		
	Environmental	Music	Voices
Relief (using soothing sound)	Sounds of nature • Waterfall • Ocean waves • Rain • Flowing water • Wind • Distant thunder • Bonfire Wildlife sounds • Birds • Crickets/ cicadas • Whales • Frogs • Jungle sounds • Island sounds Human-made sounds • White noise • Pink noise • Brown noise • Fan noise • Clothes dryer • Train	• Lullabies • Music box • Piano • Celtic music • Classical guitar • Baroque • Instrumental music • Songs in a foreign language • String quartet • Meditation music • Hypnosis music • Indian flute • Zen music • Mystical music	• Bedtime stories • Guided meditation • Guided relaxation • Soothing TED Talks • Cooking instruction • Audiobooks

Goal of Sound Therapy	Source of Sound		
	Environmental	Music	Voices
Distraction (using interesting sound)	• Bird calls • Whale songs • Dolphin communication • Wolves howling • Fox calls • Owls • Morse code	• Songs with interesting lyrics • Music that evokes positive memories • New and/ or unusual genres of music • Music with interesting instrumental parts • Baroque music	• Lectures • Audiobooks • Podcasts • Talk radio • Telephone conversations • TED Talks
Habituation (using background sound)	• Any of the sounds listed above (environmental sound for soothing sound) • Any low-level (soft) sound that is easily ignored	• Any of the sounds listed above (music for soothing sound) • Any low-level (soft) music that is easily ignored	• Crowd noise • Restaurant/ cafeteria noise • Boring lectures, audiobooks, podcasts

There are many styles of music, which can involve both musical instruments and singing, instruments only, or voices only. It can be slow-paced, fast-paced, or anything in between. Music is a very personal thing—we all have our preferences. The important thing for the person with bothersome tinnitus is that music can serve as soothing sound, interesting sound, and/or background sound.

Use of the human voice can accomplish a sense of relief from tinnitus (soothing sound), distraction from tinnitus (interesting sound), or make tinnitus less noticeable (background sound). As for environmental sounds and music, Table 9-3 provides examples of how voices can be used as soothing sound, interesting sound, and/or background sound.

Developing a Sound Plan

We just covered the information that is provided to patients to understand the numerous ways that sound can be used as therapy for bothersome tinnitus. We will now talk about how that information is used to design specific uses of sound to address situations in which tinnitus is bothersome. We refer to this as *developing a sound plan*. We use a worksheet to assist in this process—the Sound Plan Worksheet (Fig. 9-4).

Figure 9-4. The Sound Plan Worksheet. This worksheet is used to develop a plan for how sound will be used to manage a "bothersome tinnitus situation" (#1 on the worksheet). The sound plan consists of the answers recorded for #2, #3, and #4 on the worksheet. When the plan has been used for a week or two, #5 is completed to rate how well the plan worked. Comments can be provided in #6. Note that this worksheet is used for developing a **single** sound plan. More plans can be developed as needed.

Sound Plan Worksheet

1. Write down one bothersome tinnitus situation _____

2. Check one or more of the three ways to use sound to manage the situation	3. Write down the sounds that you will try	4. Write down the devices you will use	5. Use your sound plan over the **next week. How helpful** was each sound after using it for 1 week?	6. Comments When you find something that works well (or not so well) please comment. You do not need to wait 1 week to write your comments.
☐ Soothing sound (TINNITUS)			Not at all ☐ ☐ ☐ A little ☐ ☐ ☐ Moderately ☐ ☐ ☐ Very much ☐ ☐ ☐ Extremely ☐ ☐ ☐	
☐ Background sound (TINNITUS)			Not at all ☐ ☐ ☐ A little ☐ ☐ ☐ Moderately ☐ ☐ ☐ Very much ☐ ☐ ☐ Extremely ☐ ☐ ☐	
☐ Interesting sound (TINNITUS)			Not at all ☐ ☐ ☐ A little ☐ ☐ ☐ Moderately ☐ ☐ ☐ Very much ☐ ☐ ☐ Extremely ☐ ☐ ☐	

This document is available as a free download on the Resources page at https://www.earsgonewrong.org/

119

The idea behind the Sound Plan Worksheet is for people to develop personalized sound plans. This is done by first identifying the *most bothersome tinnitus situation* that the sound plan will attempt to address. The Tinnitus Problem Checklist is used to identify the most bothersome tinnitus situation, as well as the second- and third-most bothersome tinnitus situations (Fig. 9-5).

Tinnitus Problem Checklist

1. My most bothersome tinnitus situation is:

- ☐ Falling asleep at night
- ☐ Staying asleep at night
- ☐ Waking up in the morning
- ☐ Reading
- ☐ Working at the computer
- ☐ Relaxing in my recliner
- ☐ Napping during the day
- ☐ Planning activities
- ☐ Driving
- ☐ Other _____

Now, write your answer on #1 of the Sound Plan Worksheet and/or the Changing Thoughts and Feelings Worksheet.

2. My second most bothersome tinnitus situation is:

- ☐ Falling asleep at night
- ☐ Staying asleep at night
- ☐ Waking up in the morning
- ☐ Reading
- ☐ Working at the computer
- ☐ Relaxing in my recliner
- ☐ Napping during the day
- ☐ Planning activities
- ☐ Driving
- ☐ Other _____

Now, write your answer on #1 of a *separate* worksheet.

3. My third most bothersome tinnitus situation is:

- ☐ Falling asleep at night
- ☐ Staying asleep at night
- ☐ Waking up in the morning
- ☐ Reading
- ☐ Working at the computer
- ☐ Relaxing in my recliner
- ☐ Napping during the day
- ☐ Planning activities
- ☐ Driving
- ☐ Other _____

Now, write your answer on #1 of a *separate* worksheet.

This document is available as a free download on the Resources page at https://www.earsgonewrong.org/

Figure 9-5. The Tinnitus Problem Checklist. This checklist is used to identify a person's *most bothersome tinnitus situation*, which can be any of the problem areas listed as response choices. Whatever the *most bothersome* tinnitus situation is, that situation is addressed first by developing a *plan* to manage that situation (using either the Sound Plan Worksheet or the Changing Thoughts and Feelings Worksheet). The Checklist also includes items to identify the *second-* and *third-most bothersome* tinnitus situations. Any situation that is impacted by tinnitus can be identified and separate plans developed to manage that specific situation.

Developing a sound plan always starts by identifying the *most bothersome* tinnitus situation as identified on the Tinnitus Problem Checklist. Whatever that is, it is entered as item #1 in the Sound Plan Worksheet. The next three items (#2, #3, and #4) on the Sound Plan Worksheet are the actual sound plan that will be used for the purpose of making the most bothersome tinnitus situation *less bothersome.*

The most common tinnitus-related problem is sleep disturbance—either falling asleep when going to bed or staying asleep throughout the night. For example, if "falling asleep at night" is checked as the most bothersome tinnitus situation on the Tinnitus Problem Checklist, then a sound plan will be developed to assist in specifically helping the person fall asleep. The

> Developing a sound plan always starts by identifying the *most bothersome* tinnitus situation as identified on the Tinnitus Problem Checklist.

sound plan starts with #2 on the Sound Plan Worksheet by identifying which of the three approaches to using sound (soothing, interesting, and/or background) might work for this purpose.

Next is #3 on the Sound Plan Worksheet where specific sounds are listed that will be used to address the most bothersome tinnitus situation. Table 9-3 can be a good starting point for selecting sounds that will be used for this purpose. Many examples are provided for each of the nine combinations of sounds that are on the sound grid. Once the specific sounds are selected, then devices that will be the sources of the sounds will be selected for #4.

To summarize, the tinnitus problem to be addressed with the sound plan is #1 on the Sound Plan Worksheet. The sound plan itself is whatever is selected for #2, #3, and #4. For #2, three approaches to using sound can be chosen to meet different objectives—soothing sound for relief, interesting sound for distraction, and background sound for habituation. Once those objectives are established, then specific sounds are chosen for each and #3 is filled out with those sounds. Finally, #4 is used to select devices that will be used as sources of the sounds that were chosen in #3. That's the sound plan that will be used for a week or two and then evaluated in #5—each sound chosen is rated as "not at all," "a little," "moderately," "very much," or "extremely" helpful. Any comments can be entered in #6. An example of how "Bob" filled out the Sound Plan Worksheet is shown in Figure 9-6.

Figure 9-6. Example of "Bob's" Sound Plan Worksheet. For #1, the bothersome tinnitus situation he chose to work on was "falling asleep at night." For #2, he selected the sound therapy approach of using background sound (to make his tinnitus less noticeable) and interesting sound (to distract him from thinking about his tinnitus). For #3, the specific sounds he intended to use were fan noise (as background sound) and television, a favorite podcast, and an audiobook (all as interesting sound). For #4, the devices he intended to use as the source of the sounds were a box fan (for background sound), the TV in his bedroom, a smartphone with earbuds, and a radio by the bed with earbuds (all for interesting sound). He used this plan (#2, #3, and #4) for a week and then completed #5 to rate how helpful each sound was. The fan noise was "moderately" helpful. The TV was "a little" helpful. The smartphone with earbuds was "very much" helpful, and the radio by the bed with earbuds was "not at all" helpful. He wrote comments about each in #6.

Bob

Sound Plan Worksheet

1. Write down one bothersome tinnitus situation _falling asleep at night_

2. Check one or more of the three ways to use sound to manage the situation

3. Write down the sounds that you will try

4. Write down the devices you will use

5. Use your sound plan over the next week. How helpful was each sound after using it for 1 week?

6. Comments
When you find something that works well (or not so well) please comment. You do not need to wait 1 week to write your comments.

Section	Sounds	Devices	Not at all	A little	Moderately	Very much	Extremely	Comments
☐ **Soothing sound** (TINNITUS)			☐	☐	☐	☐	☐	
			☐	☐	☐	☐	☐	
☒ **Background sound** (TINNITUS)	fan	box fan	☐	☐	☒	☐	☐	_adding fan noise helped me get to sleep and_
			☐	☐	☐	☐	☐	_helped me stay asleep_
☒ **Interesting sound** (TINNITUS)	television	TV in bedroom	☒	☐	☐	☐	☐	
	podcast	smartphone with earbuds	☐	☒	☐	☒	☐	_the podcast helped me get to sleep but I still_
	audiobook	radio with earbuds	☐	☐	☐	☐	☐	_wake up in the night_

Summary of Level 3 Skills Education: Sound Therapy

We've completed the basic instruction about individualized sound therapy that is provided by audiologists. This information can be provided in a single session. It's important, however, to have a follow-up session to evaluate how well the person's sound plan worked and to reinforce using it on an ongoing basis. The Sound Plan Worksheet is not intended to be used just once. Rather, it is intended to be used as often and as long as necessary to learn which sounds and sound-delivering devices are most effective in accomplishing the desired sound therapy goals.

> It's important...to have a follow-up session to evaluate how well the person's sound plan worked and to reinforce using it on an ongoing basis.

Sound Therapy: Test Your Knowledge

Please read each statement and then circle the one best answer.

1. The main goal of using soothing sound is to:
   a. make you feel better as soon as you hear it
   b. shift your attention away from your tinnitus
   c. reduce contrast to make it easier to ignore your tinnitus
   d. make your tinnitus quieter

2. The main goal of using background sound is to:
   a. make you feel better as soon as you hear it
   b. shift your attention away from your tinnitus
   c. reduce contrast to make it easier to ignore your tinnitus
   d. make your tinnitus quieter

3. The main goal of using interesting sound is to:
   a. make you feel better as soon as you hear it
   b. shift your attention away from your tinnitus
   c. reduce contrast to make it easier to ignore your tinnitus
   d. make your tinnitus quieter

4. Which of these is a goal of tinnitus management?
   a. cure tinnitus
   b. reduce emotional reactions
   c. make tinnitus quieter
   d. make tinnitus go away

5. Your Sound Plan Worksheet should be used:
   a. only once, without making changes
   b. to plan how to use sound when tinnitus is a problem
   c. to plan how to use sound to make tinnitus quieter
   d. to plan how to use sound to help you hear better

6. Background sound:
   a. is so soft you almost can't hear it
   b. is always white noise
   c. might not help right away, but can help long-term
   d. is soothing sound

7. The Sound Plan Worksheet:
   a. requires the use of soothing sound
   b. can be used over and over
   c. does not include wearable listening devices
   d. should not be changed once it's completed

8. The "candle in a dark room" is used to explain why:
   a. soothing sound can be helpful
   b. interesting sound can be helpful
   c. background sound can be helpful
   d. annoying sound is not helpful

9. Voices can be used as
   a. interesting sound only
   b. interesting sound and/or background sound
   c. interesting sound and/or soothing sound
   d. soothing sound, interesting sound, and/or background sound

10. If your tinnitus bothers you at night, which of these might help you sleep?
    a. soothing sound
    b. background sound
    c. interesting sound
    d. all of the above

Answer key: 1=a; 2=c; 3=b; 4=b; 5=b; 6=c; 7=b; 8=c; 9=d; 10=d

CHAPTER 10

Level 3 Skills Education: Cognitive Behavioral Therapy

Goals of CBT in General

The overall goal of CBT is to improve a person's health.[162] Treatment with CBT is intended to change behaviors and thoughts to *decrease emotional reactions* to a physical or mental health condition and *increase the ability to function normally* in life (with respect to sleep, concentration, relationships, etc.). To conduct CBT, the clinician can draw from an assortment of treatment strategies (different approaches to treatment). Each strategy uses a different path to achieve its goals.[51] The strategies are either "cognitive" or "behavioral"—in accordance with the name *cognitive behavioral therapy*.

Clinicians have different priorities with respect to their choice of the CBT treatment strategies that are available.

In addition, other forms of psychological treatment can be integrated into the CBT protocol, such as acceptance and commitment therapy (ACT) and mindfulness therapies (that go by different names).[51] There is considerable variability in how CBT is practiced across different practitioners.

Adaptation of CBT to Treat Tinnitus

CBT was originally used to treat pain, anxiety, depression, and insomnia and was later adapted to treat tinnitus.[50,170,171] It was first described as a treatment for tinnitus by the audiologist Dr. Robert Sweetow at the University of California, San Francisco.[172,173] CBT-for-tinnitus was later described by numerous investigators[50,99] and is currently not associated with any particular individual or group.

> CBT was originally used to treat pain, anxiety, depression, and insomnia and was later adapted to treat tinnitus.

A working assumption is "What is good for life in general is usually good for coping with tinnitus. This includes living a healthy life with respect to food, exercise, social contacts, and so on."[174] (p. 99) With that assumption in mind, CBT is based on the foundational principle that behaviors, thoughts, and emotions are interconnected—changing one of these tends to change the others.[62]

According to systematic reviews and clinical practice guidelines that have been published, CBT has the "strongest research evidence" of all available tinnitus treatments.[14,87,88,175] It has even been delivered as an online program with reportedly good results.[176,177] In spite of its glowing reputation, CBT has not been proven to be superior to other established methods of treatment for tinnitus (described in chapter 3).

> CBT is based on the foundational principle that behaviors, thoughts, and emotions are interconnected— changing one of these tends to change the others.

Goals of CBT for Treating Tinnitus

For treating tinnitus with CBT, the objective of the *cognitive* approach is to identify thoughts and beliefs about tinnitus that are negative and replace them with thoughts and beliefs that are constructive.[65] This strategy is referred to as *cognitive restructuring*. For PTM, we refer to cognitive restructuring as *changing thoughts*.

The objective of the *behavioral* approach is to engage in activities and learn coping skills that counter the emotional and functional effects of tinnitus.[65] The treatment strategies generally include distraction activities, making behavioral changes, learning relaxation methods, and making lifestyle changes to improve sleep and to optimize auditory and overall health. Certain strategies are thought to be more helpful than others for treating tinnitus.[51] These will be discussed further below.

Which Clinicians Perform CBT?

CBT is most commonly performed by psychologists but also by other psychological health providers (clinical social workers, advanced nurse practitioners, professional counselors, psychiatrists).[178] Although providers may have expertise in CBT, very few are proficient in delivering CBT *for the management of tinnitus.*[162] This creates a conundrum: CBT is reported to have the strongest research evidence for treating tinnitus, and yet very few providers offer CBT specifically for tinnitus.[62]

> Although providers may have expertise in CBT, very few are proficient in delivering CBT *for the management of tinnitus.*

A partial solution to this conundrum has been proposed by tinnitus researchers and clinicians.[62,178] They pointed out that providers outside of the psychological health arena have administered CBT successfully to treat depression, social anxiety disorder, generalized anxiety disorder, and panic disorder. It therefore seems reasonable that audiologists, who are most commonly contacted by people seeking clinical services for tinnitus, could administer CBT. "It seems evident that audiologists can at least provide certain components of CBT without extensive training. . . . Audiologists can offer a viable pathway for expanding tinnitus management services in populations in which psychological health providers are not readily available."[178] (p. 287)

Audiologists and other non-psychological health clinicians should not perform CBT without receiving proper training and supervision.[178] The *behavioral* components of CBT, which mostly involve relaxation and distraction techniques, require much less training than the *cognitive* components. Patients would have greater access to research-based tinnitus treatment if audiologists (and other non-psychological health clinicians) were to learn to teach at least the behavioral components.

Addition of CBT to PTM

We originally developed PTM as a method conducted entirely by audiologists (with the exception of any needed referrals).[179] Our focus was to use sound therapy, as described in the previous chapter, almost exclusively. We soon realized that treatment should include CBT because even back then CBT was reported to have the strongest scientific evidence for treating tinnitus.[161] The CBT procedures described in this chapter were developed by psychologist Caroline Schmidt, PhD.[82,97,98] The addition of CBT made the PTM treatment multidisciplinary (audiology and psychological health).

The different ways CBT is delivered in the clinic vary considerably.[51,174] Treatment sessions can be conducted individually or in groups, with as few as 3 sessions or as many as 20. The length of each session is usually an hour or an hour and a half. For PTM Level 3 Skills Education it was decided to limit CBT to certain treatment strategies delivered over three 1.5-hour sessions. As we will discuss in chapter 13, delivering more strategies and more sessions of CBT are options during Level 5 Individualized Support.

Changing Thoughts—the Cognitive Approach to Treatment with CBT

The cognitive approach to treatment with CBT is based most generally on the concept that people's thoughts (*cognitions*) affect their feelings *(emotions)*.[97] What we *think* about people and events determines how we *feel* about them. And our *emotions* affect our *health*.[168] It is therefore important to assess our thoughts about tinnitus to determine if they are a primary reason tinnitus is bothersome. If so, then our thoughts might be described as "thought errors."[63] We will discuss 12 common thought errors along with how they affect our reactions to tinnitus.[97] The goal is to learn to avoid negative thinking and make our thoughts constructive toward reducing the effects of tinnitus.[62]

What we refer to as *thought errors* are also referred to as *cognitive distortions, negative cognitions,* and *automatic thoughts*.[50] They all mean essentially the same thing: thoughts that are automatic, accepted without question, and believed to be uncontrollable. Not all automatic thoughts are negative, and in fact many are positive.

> The goal is to learn to avoid negative thinking and make our thoughts constructive toward reducing the effects of tinnitus.

We are focused here on negative thinking, which is the concern with having thought errors about tinnitus that can cause it to be a problem in many ways.

The A-B-C Model

It is important to understand the relationship between thoughts and emotions, which is most easily explained by the A-B-C model.[50]

- **A = Situation** (situation or event experienced by the person)
- **B = Thought** (thoughts, beliefs, and perceptions triggered by the situation)
- **C = Emotion** (emotional response to the thought triggered by the situation)

As an example of the A-B-C model, imagine that you've invited friends over for dinner. They were supposed to arrive at 6:00 p.m. It's now 7:00 p.m. The dinner is getting cold and they have not contacted you. Their unexplained absence is the *situation* (A), which triggers *thoughts* (B) on your part. You might think your friends were rude and selfish, which causes you to be *angry* (C). Or maybe you think they might have gotten into an accident, which makes you *worried* (C) about their welfare. Any emotions you have (C) will depend on your thoughts (B) in response to the situation (A). Importantly, "the emotional response (C) is a result of thought content (B) and not of the event itself."[50] (p. 69)

With the A-B-C model in mind, it is helpful to consider non-tinnitus situations and how any emotional responses are due to the thoughts that result from the situations.[50] Some examples of events that typically result in negative emotions are being stuck in traffic or behind a slow-moving car, spilling a glass of milk, forgetting an important appointment, or not being invited to a party. These types of situations can be discussed along with the likely emotional responses. Then, the thoughts that result in the negative emotions are analyzed along with alternative thoughts that might result in more positive emotions.

The next step is to consider sounds in the environment and how they might cause emotional responses.[50] Imagine you are sleeping at night and are awakened by a sound. The sound is the event (A), which may cause fear (C) if you think there is an intruder in your house (B). It may cause annoyance (C) if you think that wind caused the noise (B). Or it might result in a sense of relief (C) if you realize your daughter has returned home from a date (B). Most sounds in the environment do not elicit a response, but some do—especially those that get your attention. You can think about what kinds of sounds cause you to have emotional reactions and how your interpretation of the sounds causes the reactions.

Now you're ready to think about your *tinnitus as the event* (A) that can provoke thoughts (B) and emotional reactions (C).[50] It is helpful to think about the tinnitus (A) as unchanging and how thinking about it differently (B) can result in different reactions (C). We will now list 12 common thought errors, which were developed by Dr. Schmidt and included in the PTM self-help workbook.[97]

1. All-or-Nothing Thinking

Definition: When you see things in only two categories such as black or white.

Example of unhelpful thought: "Nothing I ever do is right."

Example of unhelpful tinnitus thought: "If my tinnitus is loud when I wake up in the morning, I know I will have a bad day."

Alternative (more helpful) tinnitus thought: "I'm learning ways to have a good day even when my tinnitus is loud."

2. Oversimplifying

Definition: When you see one bad event as a pattern that never changes.

Example of unhelpful thought: You get on the wrong train one time and think, "I'll never learn how to use the subway."

Example of unhelpful tinnitus thought: "I was awake all night from my tinnitus. This will happen every night."

Alternative (more helpful) tinnitus thought: "Last night my tinnitus kept me awake, but most nights I eventually fall asleep."

3. Focusing on Wrong Details

Definition: When you pick out a single detail and focus on it. You don't think about other, more positive details.

Example of unhelpful thought: "I got a 60% on my math home-work. I'm a terrible student."

Example of unhelpful tinnitus thought: "My tinnitus made it hard to enjoy dinner with a friend."

Alternative (more helpful) tinnitus thought: "My tinnitus was really loud at dinner. However, it was great to see my friend again and to catch up."

4. Jumping to Conclusions

Definition: When you think an event was unpleasant even though there are no facts to support that. You might assume that you know what someone else is thinking or that things will turn out badly.

Example of unhelpful thought: "If I go to the party then I won't know anyone and will not have fun."

Example of unhelpful tinnitus thought: "My tinnitus kept me awake last night. The next day I met a friend for coffee. I was really tired and didn't talk much. I'll bet he thought I was boring."

Alternative (more helpful) tinnitus thought: "It was difficult to be so tired all day. I told my friend about my tinnitus keeping me awake. He was very supportive."

5. Overestimating

Definition: When you think things are more important than they really are (such as your goof-up or someone else's success).

Example of unhelpful thought: "She turned me down when I asked her to go on a date with me. I don't know how to talk to women. I'll be alone forever."

Example of unhelpful tinnitus thought: "My tinnitus makes me moody. No one wants to be around me."

Alternative (more helpful) tinnitus thought: "Sometimes I'm moody and other times I am in a great mood. I have friends who know me and understand me."

6. Underestimating

Definition: When you think things are *less* important than they really are (such as your success or someone else's faults).

Example of unhelpful thought: "I know I got a 95% on the test, but I could have done better."

Example of unhelpful tinnitus thought: "I know I learned how to get to sleep even though my tinnitus is loud. I also started using soothing sound for my tinnitus at work. Even so, I'll never learn to deal with my tinnitus."

Alternative (more helpful) tinnitus thought: "I can deal with my tinnitus by making small changes. It may not be gone, but I don't notice my tinnitus as often."

7. Assuming the Worst

Definition: When you think something is much worse than it really is.

Example of unhelpful thought: A woman who got a low grade on a quiz thinks it's the end of her college career.

Example of unhelpful tinnitus thought: "I'm going to become deaf from my tinnitus."

Alternative (more helpful) tinnitus thought: "My doctor said tinnitus won't make me deaf. It just feels strange to hear this ringing in my ears all the time and not know why."

8. Emotional Thoughts

Definition: When you think that your emotions show the way things really are. You might think, "I feel it, so it must be true."

Example of unhelpful thought: "I feel like I'm the only one who cleans up around here, so you must not be helping."

Example of unhelpful tinnitus thought: "I feel like no one knows what I am going through with my tinnitus. I feel all alone."

Alternative (more helpful) tinnitus thought: "People will understand what I am going through when I explain tinnitus to them."

9. "Should" Statements

Definition: When you say "should" and "shouldn't" to try to get yourself to do hard tasks. These statements tend to make you feel guilty. (Also included are statements with the words "must" and "ought.")

Example of unhelpful thought: "I should eat healthier and stop eating food I like."

Example of unhelpful tinnitus thought: "I should not have to deal with tinnitus during the best years of my life."

Alternative (more helpful) tinnitus thought: "Tinnitus isn't what I expected when I retired, but I can deal with it."

10. Labeling

Definition: Attaching a bad label to yourself or others.

Example of unhelpful thought: "He lost his keys, so he's stupid."

Example of unhelpful tinnitus thought: "I can't deal with my tinnitus so I'm a weak person."

Alternative (more helpful) tinnitus thought: "Sometimes it's hard to deal with my tinnitus. I do my best to stay healthy and active. I practice methods for managing my reactions to tinnitus that I learned from PTM. However, sometimes the tinnitus still bothers me. That is normal."

11. Making Things Personal

Definition: You see yourself as the cause of some negative event when you are not responsible. You ignore other details.

Example of unhelpful thought: "My doctor was not nice to me because I was sick."

Example of unhelpful tinnitus thought: "My tinnitus made it hard for me to enjoy the picnic. I caused everyone else to have a bad time too."

Alternative (more helpful) tinnitus thought: "My tinnitus made it hard for me to enjoy the picnic. No one can have fun all of the time."

12. Blaming

Definition: You blame others for your problems. You may also blame yourself for other people's problems.

Example of unhelpful thought: "I didn't get the job because you didn't call to give me a pep talk before my meeting."

Example of unhelpful tinnitus thought: "My tinnitus wouldn't be a problem if my wife was more supportive."

Alternative (more helpful) tinnitus thought: "It would be helpful if my wife was more supportive. Either way I would have to work at dealing with my tinnitus."

Changing thoughts to feel better may seem straightforward, but it is often challenging for people to purposely change their thoughts from what they're used to. Just learning the process of changing thoughts is likely inadequate for most people to be successful with this technique. I mentioned that we limited the number of CBT sessions to three for PTM Level 3 Skills Education, which has been referred to as *brief CBT*.[65] That is a bare-bones approach to teach the basic cognitive and behavioral techniques. Normally, more sessions are needed, and it has been recommended that at least eight sessions may be required to be most successful with CBT.[50]

If you are motivated to try changing your thoughts on your own, I'm providing some tips below that come from the PTM self-help workbook[97] and two landmark books describing CBT for tinnitus.[50,180] Of course, the ideal is to work with a CBT provider who is skilled in teaching these techniques.

Let's start with the situation, or event, which is your perception of the tinnitus sensation (A in the A-B-C model). The situation/event can also be experiences you have that are associated with your tinnitus. For example, going to bed at night may be the time when you are most aware of your tinnitus, and you struggle to get to sleep. While lying in bed you might think, "This sound is driving me crazy—I'm never going to get to sleep." That thought (B) results in anger, frustration, and anxiety (C). This kind of thinking and reacting might be a habit every time you go to bed. What can you do?

The reactions (C) are the problem, and they are triggered by the thoughts (B). So the key is to *change the thoughts in such a way that the reactions become more positive*. It may not seem possible, but we do have control over our thoughts. We have to believe that this is possible, and then it takes practice (probably lots of practice) to make our "automatic thoughts" more positive. How can that be done using our example, "This sound is driving me crazy—I'm never going to get to sleep"? That is the natural (or habitual) thought that creates the problem. Three techniques can be used to interrupt and control this type of negative thought: thought-stopping, distraction, and increasing positive thoughts.[180]

Thought-Stopping

When you notice the negative thought, *immediately* do one or more of the following:[180]

- Think to yourself, "I'm going to stop thinking about that right now."
- Imagine a stoplight turning from yellow to red, which says you *have to* stop the thought.
- Shout (in your mind) "Stop!" Imagine that it is a command you must obey.
- Wear a rubber band on your wrist and snap it when you think the negative thought. (People report this actually works!)
- Taking a deep breath, think the word *One*. Then think the word *Relax* while you breathe out slowly and relax all the muscles in your body.

Distraction

This technique is done immediately after thought-stopping.[180] You interrupted the negative thought, and now you want to focus on a non-negative thought. The key here is to focus on a thought that keeps your attention. Here are some suggestions for how to do that:[180]

- In your mind count backward from 100. This should be moderately challenging, such as counting by three (for example, 100, 97, 94, 91 . . .).
- In your mind recite the alphabet backwards (z, y, x, w, v, . . .).
- In your mind list the months backward (December, November, October, . . .).
- In your mind recite the words to a familiar song.
- Think about the details of your last (enjoyable) holiday.
- Imagine how you would spend a million dollars.
- Imagine a favorite place and how it affects all your senses.
- Create a shopping list.
- Plan a menu for an extravagant dinner.
- Think about a movie you enjoyed.
- Plan your next holiday or birthday celebration.

Increasing Positive Thoughts

This is a general technique that would address any negative thinking. Many people are prone to focus on negative aspects of their lives (failures, regrets, tinnitus, etc.) rather than positive aspects (successes, achievements, good friends, enjoyable hobbies, etc.). Shifting thoughts from negative to positive is not an easy process, but it is definitely doable with sustained effort. Here are two suggestions to assist with this process:[180]

> Shifting thoughts from negative to positive is not an easy process, but it is definitely doable with sustained effort.

First, purchase a small spiral notebook (such as 3x5 inches) that you can carry with you. On each page write down something positive about yourself. If you have trouble with this, ask family and friends to tell you positive things about yourself and write them down. Get in the habit of looking at one page in the notebook and focusing intently on the positive thought written on it. When the notebook is open, add anything positive you think of on blank pages. If you can make this a regular habit, it will eventually change your usual thinking to be more positive.

Second, you can pair positive thinking with different events during the day: when you first get up in the morning, when you brush your teeth, when you eat, before you go to bed at night, etc. Create reminders for yourself so that the events serve as triggers to remind you to think a positive thought.

We're just scratching the surface regarding the process of learning to think about tinnitus more positively and constructively. For example, we have not discussed the important recommendation to challenge negative thoughts using a step-by-step approach. Three self-help books are available to assist in this effort.[62,97,180] Each of these books contains much more detail than what we've covered here. But, again, working with a CBT specialist is the most effective way to learn these techniques.

Changing Behaviors—the Behavioral Approach to Treatment with CBT

Regarding the behavioral approach for CBT, the treatment is based most generally on the concept that changing our behavior in certain ways can make tinnitus less of a problem. Common *behavioral* strategies that are used with CBT-for-tinnitus are *practicing relaxation exercises* and *increasing pleasant activities*.[97] Additional behavioral strategies include *addressing sleep problems* and *enriching the sound environment*.[62] All of these behavioral strategies are intended to promote participation in positive and pleasant activities, shifting attention away from tinnitus whenever it is bothersome, and using stress-reduction techniques.

In addition, CBT provides information about tinnitus (its characteristics, causes, effects, etc.) and hearing loss—most of this information was covered in chapter 2, which is more fully described in my general book about tinnitus.[4] We are now going to focus on the behavioral strategies that are taught during PTM Level 3 Skills Education. These strategies include two relaxation exercises (*deep breathing* and *imagery*) and activities to "help you enjoy life and pay less attention to your tinnitus"[97] [(p. 44)] (referred to as *planning pleasant activities*).

Relaxation Exercises

It is common for people with tinnitus to report that feeling stressed makes their tinnitus worse. It can be difficult to determine, however, whether stress makes tinnitus worse or tinnitus worsens (or causes) stress.

We intuitively know what stress is, but it would take a whole book to describe what goes on in the body when stress is experienced. To simplify things, we'll just briefly mention the *fight-or-flight response* and *chronic stress.*

Sensing danger or being fearful causes changes in the body that prepare it for fight-or-flight.[168] These changes include shutdown of digestive functions, release of adrenaline into the blood, and increases in heart rate, breathing rate, and muscle tension. Fight-or-flight is the highest level of stress and cannot be sustained for very long. If these changes in the body are not strong enough to induce the fight-or-flight response, they still cause stress. Stress that is chronic can cause anxiety, exhaustion, sleep deprivation, and trouble concentrating.

Many sources of stress can affect a person at the same time—the stress a person experiences is the combination of all these sources. Tinnitus just adds to the stress. It may add only slightly, or it may be the primary contributor. Regardless, if a person feels stressed, it is important to reduce the stress, which is the purpose of the relaxation exercises that are used with CBT. We will now discuss those exercises—deep breathing and imagery.

Deep breathing means *focusing on your breathing to help you relax.*[97] Imagery means *imagining a calming and peaceful place.* Both of these exercises can calm your body, focus your mind away from the tinnitus, and help you feel more relaxed. Ultimately, these exercises can bring relief from tension and stress caused by tinnitus and help you think more clearly, function better, and feel better overall.

Preparing to do Relaxation Exercises

If you are going to try either deep breathing or imagery, you would start by finding a place that is quiet where you will not be disturbed.[97] Your clothing should be loose, and the room temperature should be comfortable. Sit in a comfortable chair with your feet propped up or flat on the floor—whichever you prefer. Turn on some sound that is soothing. Background sound can also suffice. (Soothing and background sound are defined in chapter 9.) You want to avoid silence because of the tendency to focus on the tinnitus when it is the only "sound." (See the contrast reduction section in chapter 9.)

Deep Breathing

While sitting comfortably in your chair, place one hand on your chest and one hand on your stomach.[97] Breathe in normally and notice which hand rises the most. It will probably be the one on your chest, which shows that you are breathing shallow breaths from your lungs. Now take a breath *from your stomach*, which will first expand your stomach and then expand your chest. That's what deep breathing is.

Now either close your eyes or look at one object in the room.[97] Take a deep breath through your nose (breathing from your stomach) and count slowly from one to three. Hold that breath for about two seconds and then exhale from your mouth, counting from one to three. That's the exercise, and it should be repeated at least five times.

When done, count back very slowly from three to one.[97] When you say "three," become aware of your surroundings. When you say "two," move your hands, arms, feet, and legs, and turn your head back and forth. When you say "one," open your eyes and think about how relaxed you feel.

Imagery

As described, you are sitting comfortably in your chair. You are going to choose a place (imaginary or real) that is calming and peaceful and feels safe to you.[97] It might be the beach, a garden, or even your kitchen. Think about your five senses when choosing this peaceful place. What do you *see*? What do you *hear*? What do you *feel* touching your body? What are the *smells* in the air? Can you *taste* anything?

Now that you are imagining your peaceful place, imagine walking slowly through that place. While you're walking, what do you see, hear, feel, smell, and taste? Reach out and touch the things that are around you. Keep digging deeper into the image. You should feel calm and peaceful. Be aware of how your body feels so that you can remember this feeling next time you do the imagery exercise. When you're ready to stop, count down from three to one in the same way as described for ending the deep breathing exercise.

Planning Pleasant Activities

Pleasant activities are things you *like* to do but are not *required* to do.[97] Their purpose is to give you more positive feelings, distract you from thinking about your tinnitus, and help you feel better overall.

Some people feel that their tinnitus makes it impossible to enjoy life.[97] Because of this, they may stop doing activities they normally would enjoy. Doing fewer enjoyable activities in turn causes them to focus more on their tinnitus. Focusing more on tinnitus has a cascading effect of reacting emotionally and having trouble sleeping and concentrating.

> Pleasant activities are things you like to do but are not *required* to do.

The cascade of effects that occur when focusing more on tinnitus can be at least partially reversed by engaging in enjoyable activities *even when your tinnitus is bothersome.*[97] Engaging in pleasant activities can help you pay less attention to the tinnitus, react to it less, and enjoy life more.

Because of your tinnitus, it might be difficult to enjoy activities that used to be enjoyable. It might feel like you're having to relearn how to have the same level of enjoyment you once had. It takes extra effort to overcome this hurdle. Over time, however, you should once again be able to enjoy your favorite activities.

People generally wait until they feel good to engage in a fun activity. If we are constantly reacting to tinnitus, then it may be a long wait before we "feel good." If you let your feelings determine what you do, you may end up just staying home and feeling discouraged. To increase the number of enjoyable activities, it is therefore important to *plan ahead.*[97] By planning ahead, you put these activities on your calendar and your feelings should not stop you from doing them.

It is also important to keep track of your activities to help you become more aware of how you spend each day.[97] It is helpful to think of two categories of activities: things you are *required to do,* and things you *like to do but are not required to do.* It takes effort, but tracking your activities can be very revealing about how you spend your time. If the required tasks far outnumber the enjoyable activities, then it's important to put more pleasant activities on your calendar.

It can be helpful to make a list of 10 activities you would enjoy.[97] These can all be activities you do by yourself or with other people. The types of activities can be categorized using the categories listed in Table 10-1. From your list, schedule activities to your calendar at specific times each day. Start with one per day, and write down how long you will do the activity.

Table 10-1. Categories of Pleasant Activities with Examples of Each.[97,180]

Type of Activity	Example Activity	Your Activity
Artistic	Draw or paint	
Collecting	Collect old lanterns	
Cooking	Try new recipes	

Type of Activity	Example Activity	Your Activity
Creative	Write poetry or a short story	
Educational	Watch a documentary	
Musical	Learn to play the ukulele	
Pampering	Go to a spa	
Recreational	Take dance lessons	
Social	Meet friends for coffee	
Solitary	Take a nature walk	
Sporting	Play Ping-Pong or pickleball	
Travel	Go somewhere new	

Finally, evaluate how much you enjoyed each activity that you planned.[97] You can note your assessment on each entry in your calendar—even writing a number from 1 (least enjoyable) to 10 (most enjoyable) will be helpful. Questions you can ask yourself include:

- Did I notice my tinnitus less when I did this activity?
- Would more activities be helpful?
- Am I doing all the activities that I scheduled? If not, why not?

The Changing Thoughts and Feelings Worksheet

We've covered three CBT skills: changing thoughts, relaxation exercises, and planning pleasant activities. To apply these skills in an effort to reduce the effects of tinnitus, my research group developed the Changing Thoughts and Feelings Worksheet (Fig. 10-1).[97] The worksheet is designed to help you create a plan of action for how you intend to change your thoughts and feelings about your tinnitus—using any or all of the three CBT skills.

Figure 10-1. The Changing Thoughts and Feelings Worksheet. This worksheet is used to develop a plan for how CBT skills will be used to manage a "bothersome tinnitus situation" (#1 on the worksheet). The plan itself consists of what is filled in for #2 and #3 on the worksheet. When the plan has been used for a week or two, #4 is completed to rate how well the plan worked. Comments can be written in #5. Note that this worksheet is used for developing a *single* CBT skills plan. More plans can be developed as needed. This process continues until any plans used are considered effective for reducing effects of tinnitus.

Changing Thoughts and Feelings Worksheet

1. From the Tinnitus Problem Checklist, write down one bothersome tinnitus situation. _____

2. Check one or more of the three skills to manage the situation

3. Write down the details for each skill you will use

5. Use your plan over the next week. How helpful was each exercise?

6. Comments Comments When you find something that works well (or not so well) please comment. You do not need to wait 1 week to write your comments.

☐ **Relaxation exercises**

[Relax — breathe / imagine]

☐ Deep breathing

☐ Imagery

☐ Other _____

	Not at all	A little	Moderately	Very much	Extremely
	☐	☐	☐	☐	☐
	☐	☐	☐	☐	☐
	☐	☐	☐	☐	☐

☐ **Plan pleasant activities**

[Pleasant activities: golf, write, walk, dance, paint]

Activity 1 _____

Activity 2 _____

Activity 3 _____

	Not at all	A little	Moderately	Very much	Extremely
	☐	☐	☐	☐	☐
	☐	☐	☐	☐	☐
	☐	☐	☐	☐	☐

☐ **Changing thoughts**

[Think → Feel]

Old _____

New _____

	Not at all	A little	Moderately	Very much	Extremely
	☐	☐	☐	☐	☐

This document is available as a free download on the Resources page at https://www.earsgonewrong.org/

As in the Sound Plan Worksheet (Fig. 9-4), the Changing Thoughts and Feelings Worksheet (Fig. 10-1) starts by identifying the *most bothersome tinnitus situation* that will be addressed with the CBT skills plan. The Tinnitus Problem Checklist (Fig. 9-5) is used to identify the most bothersome tinnitus situation, which is entered as item #1 in the Changing Thoughts and Feelings Worksheet. The next two items (#2 and #3) on the worksheet will comprise the actual plan that will be used in an attempt to make the most bothersome tinnitus situation *less bothersome.*

A common tinnitus-related problem is difficulty concentrating. For example, if "reading" is checked as the most bothersome tinnitus situation on the Tinnitus Problem Checklist (Fig. 9-5), then a CBT skills plan will be developed to assist in specifically helping the person concentrate on reading. The plan starts with #2 on the Changing Thoughts and Feelings Worksheet (Fig. 10-1) by identifying one or more of the three CBT skills (changing thoughts, relaxation exercises, planning pleasant activities) that you think might work for this purpose.

Next is #3 on the Changing Thoughts and Feelings Worksheet, "Write down the details for each skill you will use."

If "Relaxation exercises" is checked for #2, then three options are listed as the details for #3: "Deep breathing," "Imagery," and "Other."

If "Plan pleasant activities" is checked for #2, then up to three activities can be written in (Activity 1, Activity 2, Activity 3).

If "Changing thoughts" is checked for #2, then for #3 the "Old thought" is written down as well as the "New thought."

To summarize, the tinnitus-problem situation to be addressed with the CBT skills plan is #1 on the Changing Thoughts and Feelings Worksheet (Fig. 10-1). The CBT skills plan itself is whatever is selected for #2 and #3. For #2, three CBT skills can be chosen—relaxation exercises, plan pleasant activities, and changing thoughts. When the CBT skills to be tried are selected, then the details of each skill will be written down for #3. That's the CBT skills plan that will be used for a week or so and then evaluated in #4—each CBT skill chosen is rated as "not at all helpful," "a little helpful," "moderately helpful," "very much helpful," or "extremely helpful." Any comments can be written in #5.

We are going to use an example of how "Joe" completed his first Changing Thoughts and Feelings Worksheet (see Fig. 10-2). For #1, he entered "My tinnitus makes it hard for me to concentrate at work" as his most bothersome tinnitus situation. For #2, he checked all three CBT skills (relaxation exercises, plan pleasant activities, and changing thoughts) that he planned to try to help him concentrate better at work. He then wrote down for #3 the details of each of the skills he chose for #2. For relaxation exercises he chose deep breathing, imagery, and other (meditation). For plan pleasant activities he wrote "take a walk during lunch" as his only activity. For changing thoughts he wrote "I can't think about anything but my tinnitus" as his "old thought" and "There are many ways I can focus on things other than my tinnitus" as his "new thought."

Joe   Changing Thoughts and Feelings Worksheet

1. From the Tinnitus Problem Checklist, write down one bothersome tinnitus situation. _My tinnitus makes it hard for me to concentrate at work_

2. Check one or more of the three skills to manage the situation

3. Write down the details for each skill you will use

5. Use your plan over the next week. How helpful was each exercise?

6. Comments When you find something that works well (or not so well) please comment. You do not need to wait 1 week to write your comments.

☒ **Relaxation exercises**

	Not at all	A little	Moderately	Very much	Extremely	Comments
☒ Deep breathing	☐	☐	☐	☒	☐	_This helps!_
☒ Imagery	☐	☒	☐	☐	☐	_This helps a little_
☒ Other _meditation_	☐	☐	☐	☒	☐	_This feels good_

☒ **Plan pleasant activities**

	Not at all	A little	Moderately	Very much	Extremely	Comments
Activity 1 _Take a walk during lunch_	☐	☐	☒	☐	☐	_It was easier for me to concentrate after taking a walk_
Activity 2 _____	☐	☐	☐	☐	☐	
Activity 3 _____	☐	☐	☐	☐	☐	

☒ **Changing thoughts**

Old _I can't think about anything but my tinnitus_

New _There are many ways I can focus on things other than my tinnitus_

	Not at all	A little	Moderately	Very much	Extremely	Comments
	☐	☐	☒	☐	☐	_I feel better_

Figure 10-2. "Joe's" Changing Thoughts and Feelings Worksheet. For #1, the bothersome tinnitus situation he chose to work on was "My tinnitus makes it hard for me to concentrate at work." For #2, he selected all three CBT skills

to manage his bothersome tinnitus situation: relaxation exercises, plan pleasant activities, and changing thoughts. For #3, he selected deep breathing, imagery, and meditation as the details for relaxation exercises. He wrote "take a walk during lunch" as the only activity for plan pleasant activities. For changing thoughts he wrote "I can't think about anything but my tinnitus" as his "old thought" and "There are many ways I can focus on things other than my tinnitus" as his "new thought." He used this CBT skills plan (#2 and #3) for a week and then completed #4 to rate how helpful each CBT skill was. For relaxation exercises, deep breathing was "very much" helpful, imagery was "a little" helpful, and meditation was "very much" helpful. For plan pleasant activities, taking a walk during lunch was "moderately" helpful. For changing thoughts, thinking the "new thought" instead of the "old thought" was "moderately" helpful. He wrote comments about each in #5.

Summary of Level 3 Skills Education: Cognitive Behavioral Therapy

Whole books have been written describing CBT for tinnitus, and they greatly expand on the material presented here.[62,180] These books are particularly appropriate because they are written specifically for individuals who are struggling with tinnitus. They are easy to read and very comprehensive for those who wish to delve deeper into CBT for tinnitus.

The treatment described in chapter 9 (sound therapy) and chapter 10 (CBT) is what comprises PTM Level 3 Skills

> The treatment described in chapter 9 (sound therapy) and chapter 10 (CBT) is what comprises PTM Level 3 Skills Education.

Education. Normally it takes five sessions to cover all of this material. Importantly, these procedures were evaluated in two randomized controlled trials. Both trials showed good efficacy for the treatment (details can be seen in appendix A). The results of these trials provide evidence that the treatment is beneficial to the majority of individuals who receive it.

Cognitive Behavioral Therapy: Test Your Knowledge

Please read each statement and then circle the one best answer.

1. Cognitive behavioral therapy (CBT):
   a. can help change how you think and what you do to manage tinnitus
   b. is only helpful for mental health problems
   c. is only helpful for tinnitus
   d. can help change thoughts but not emotions

2. Which of these would help you reduce stress?
   a. deep breathing and imagery
   b. think of stress as a threat
   c. avoid exercise
   d. practice short and quick breathing

3. Relaxation exercises:
   a. quiet your tinnitus
   b. help you focus on your tinnitus
   c. speed up your breath and heart rate
   d. slow down your breath and heart rate

4. Deep breathing exercises:
   a. should be done in complete quiet
   b. should be done while standing
   c. involve holding your breath for 15 seconds
   d. involve slow breathing from your abdomen

5. The purpose of adding pleasant activities to your day is to:
   a. make your tinnitus quieter
   b. distract you from your tinnitus
   c. make your tinnitus go away
   d. improve your hearing

6. Thought errors are:
   a. able to make you feel better
   b. unhelpful thoughts
   c. out of your control
   d. helpful and healthy

7. Which of the following is a **corrected** thought error?
   a. Nothing I ever do is right
   b. I am a failure if I don't manage my tinnitus perfectly
   c. I am learning ways to have a good day even when my tinnitus is loud
   d. If my tinnitus is loud when I wake up, I know I will have a bad day

8. Which of the following is a **corrected** thought error?
   a. Last night my tinnitus kept me awake, but most nights I eventually fall asleep
   b. I was awake all night from tinnitus—this will happen every night
   c. I will never learn how to use my Sound Plan
   d. I will never learn how to use my Changing Thoughts and Feelings Plan

9. Before I can change my thoughts, I must first:
   a. identify thoughts I had before feeling bad
   b. listen to relaxing sounds
   c. consult with my psychological health provider
   d. practice deep breathing exercises

10. Which one of these statements is true?
    a. Thoughts affect health
    b. Feelings cannot be changed
    c. Feelings and thoughts are the same
    d. Thought errors are rare

11. Which of these statements is true?
    a. You might not notice relaxation exercises helping right away—but that does not mean they are not helping
    b. Reducing pleasant activities can help you get better at ignoring tinnitus
    c. It is best to practice relaxation exercises in a quiet environment
    d. Tinnitus is more likely to get your attention when you stay busy

12. Which of these can be a **first** step toward changing your thoughts?
    a. Picture yourself having positive thoughts in the future
    b. Identify what was going on when you started to feel bad (the event itself)
    c. Think about bad feelings you were having
    d. Think about good feelings you were having

13. The step-by-step process of changing thoughts includes:
    a. making a list of pleasant activities
    b. pairing positive thinking with different events during the day
    c. ignoring your feelings
    d. doing the relaxation exercises when you feel happy and content

14. The new positive thought should be:
    a. very detailed
    b. easy to remember
    c. what you want to think, even if you know it's not true
    d. fairly long

15. Which of these is the **last** step toward changing your thoughts?
    a. Picture yourself in the future
    b. Identify what you were thinking before you started to feel bad
    c. Think about bad feelings you were having
    d. Think about evidence against bad thoughts

Answer key: 1=a; 2=a; 3=d; 4=d; 5=b; 6=b; 7=c; 8=a; 9=a; 10=a; 11=a; 12=b; 13=b; 14=b; 15=a

CHAPTER 11

Evaluating Progress After Level 3 Skills Education

After patients have attended the Level 3 sessions, it is essential to follow up to determine whether their tinnitus needs have been met or if further services are required. The main objective of the sessions is to teach patients skills that will empower them to self-manage any negative effects of tinnitus. Two questionnaires are used to assess how well patients are doing with the skills they were taught—the One-Week Post-Treatment Survey and the Six-Week Post-Treatment Interview.

> Two questionnaires are used to assess how well patients are doing with the skills they were taught...

One-Week Post-Treatment Survey

The One-Week Post-Treatment Survey (shown in appendix B) is one of three questionnaires to assess how well patients are doing soon after they complete all of the Level 3 sessions. The other two questionnaires are the Tinnitus Functional Index and the Tinnitus and Hearing Survey—both of which were completed by patients prior to Level 3 treatment (see chapters 6 and 7). All of these questionnaires should be completed about one week after the final Level 3 session. Ideally the forms would be made available to be completed online. Otherwise, they can be mailed to patients and then returned by mail.

The combination of these questionnaires provides a clear picture of patients' progress (or lack of progress) with learning how to self-manage their reactions to tinnitus. Completing the Tinnitus Functional Index and the Tinnitus and Hearing Survey reveals any changes in effects of tinnitus since before the treatment. These two questionnaires, however, may not be sufficient because of the possibility that patients' self-perception of improvement might not be in agreement with changes in the scores on the questionnaires. In addition, it is important to evaluate whether patients are using the skills that were taught. The One-Week Post-Treatment Survey was developed to address both of these concerns.

> ...it is important to evaluate whether patients are using the skills that were taught.

The first four questions in the One-Week Post-Treatment Survey (appendix B) ask about the use of the different skills. Question 1 asks if sound is used to manage reactions to tinnitus. If so, how often is it used? If not, what are the reasons it is not used? Questions 2, 3, and 4 are similar in asking about the use of, respectively, practicing relaxation techniques (deep breathing and/or imagery), planning more pleasant activities, and changing thoughts about tinnitus.

The next four questions (5, 6, 7, and 8) ask about patients' subjective impression of improvement. Question 5 asks how they feel about their ability to *control their reactions* to tinnitus. Questions 6, 7, and 8 ask about, respectively, their ability to cope with tinnitus, their quality of life, and how bothered they are by their tinnitus—all compared to before they started the Level 3 sessions.

Questions 9 and 10 are more general. Question 9 asks patients if they would recommend the Level 3 sessions to someone else who has bothersome tinnitus. Question 10 is open-ended in asking patients to describe their overall experience learning how to manage their reactions to tinnitus.

Only three of the questions in the One-Week Post-Treatment Survey provide numerical response choices. Therefore, scoring the Survey is not possible. Its main purpose is to obtain information from patients to supplement the Tinnitus Functional Index and Tinnitus and Hearing Survey shortly after completing the Level 3 sessions.

Six-Week Post-Treatment Interview

Approximately six weeks after patients have attended their last Level 3 session, they should be contacted by a PTM clinician to administer the Six-Week Post-Treatment Interview (shown in appendix C). At this point it's important to conduct an *interview* rather than having patients complete a written or online questionnaire. This is a critical decision point to determine whether further services are needed, and it's important for the clinician and patient to have this conversation and make the decision together. Completing the Interview and making a decision should take between 15 and 30 minutes.

The Interview contains four questions that ask if the skills taught during the Level 3 sessions are being used, what is most helpful, what is least helpful, and the overall level of satisfaction. Based on the patient's responses there are five options for the patient: (1) no further treatment; (2) attend all sessions again; (3) attend some sessions again; (4) watch videos that provide content from the sessions; and (5) attend a Level 4 Interdisciplinary Evaluation (described in the next chapter). These options are listed on the Interview form to facilitate a collaborative decision with respect to the best course of action for the patient.

> The Interview contains four questions that ask if the skills taught during the Level 3 sessions are being used, what is most helpful, what is least helpful, and the overall level of satisfaction.

PART 4

Further Care— If Needed

CHAPTER 12

PTM Level 4 Interdisciplinary Evaluation

The majority of people who complete Level 3 Skills Education are satisfied that they know what to do to self-manage their tinnitus. The relatively few people who are not satisfied are advised to receive a PTM Level 4 Interdisciplinary Evaluation to determine why their tinnitus problem persists in spite of the care they received at Levels 2 and 3 and to make any necessary recommendations for further services.

The Level 4 evaluation is conducted by both a psychologist and an audiologist. They will attempt to determine why clinical services received in Levels 2 and 3 have not been successful. For each of the evaluation appointments, up to one hour is required. Note that a psychologist is needed for Level 4, but a

> The Level 4 evaluation is conducted by both a psychologist and an audiologist.

psychological health provider was needed for Level 3. That needs some explaining.

A psychological health provider is a less stigmatizing way of saying *mental health provider*. Some people are put off by the word *mental* because of its association with serious psychological illness. Tinnitus is a stressor that can *cause* anxiety, insomnia, concentration difficulties, and other functional and emotional effects. But tinnitus, and effects of tinnitus, would not be considered a "serious psychological illness."

Psychological health providers include advanced nurse practitioners, professional counselors, psychiatrists, psychologists, and social workers. Any psychological health provider who is competent in performing CBT-for-tinnitus can teach the Level 3 sessions. For Level 4, however, a psychologist is required because only psychologists are qualified to diagnose psychological conditions (psychiatrists are also qualified, but they rarely provide tinnitus care).

...tinnitus, and effects of tinnitus, would not be considered a "serious psychological illness."

Patients who attend the Level 4 evaluations have previously completed the Level 2 Audiology Evaluation, which included a medical history, hearing evaluation, and the Tinnitus and Hearing Survey (see chapter 6). Prior to the Level 3 sessions, they also completed the Tinnitus Functional Index (chapter 7). One week following the Level 3 sessions, they repeated the Tinnitus Functional Index and Tinnitus and Hearing Survey and also provided responses to the One-Week Post-Treatment Survey (chapter 11 and appendix B). Six weeks following the Level 3 sessions, one of the PTM clinicians interviewed the patient using the Six-Week Post-Treatment Interview (chapter 11 and appendix C). During that interview, or shortly thereafter, a decision was made whether the patient would receive a Level 4 Inter-disciplinary Evaluation. The following sections describe what is done during Level 4.

Repeat Written Questionnaires

The Level 4 assessment starts with patients completing the Tinnitus and Hearing Survey and the Tinnitus Functional Index. As explained in chapter 7, it is essential to pair any change in the TFI score with the patient's own impression as to whether there has been improvement. Normally, the measures will be in agreement, but sometimes they will not match up. Most important is the patient's impression, and because the patient is attending the Level 4 evalua-tion, it is assumed there has been little or no self-perceived improvement. The two questions in Figure 7-1 (Impression of Change-in-Tinnitus-Impact Questions) are used along with the Tinnitus Functional Index and the Tinnitus and Hearing Survey. All of these results are made available to both the audiologist and the psychologist who will be con-ducting the Level 4 evaluation.

Level 4 Evaluation by an Audiologist

If the patient reports any changes in hearing, the audiologist will conduct a full evaluation of hearing function. If not, then the evaluation focuses on administering the Tinnitus Interview (appendix D). Hearing aids may now be reconsidered for treatment if they have not been used to this point.

The Tinnitus Interview

The written tinnitus questionnaires are insufficient by themselves to evaluate patients who reach Level 4. A comprehensive face-to-face interview between the audiologist and patient is needed at this stage to conduct an in-depth evaluation to determine why tinnitus services to this point have not been adequate. The Tinnitus Interview was developed specifically for this purpose. It offers a uniform format for asking questions and recording responses. It can be completed in about 45 minutes, although that can vary considerably depending on the extent of the patient's problems.

The Tinnitus Interview supplements the Tinnitus Functional Index, the Tinnitus and Hearing Survey, and the Impression of Change-in-Tinnitus-Impact Questions. Results of the written questionnaires should first be reviewed with the patient. In addition, it may be helpful to review the case history from the Level 2 Audiology Evaluation, which would have obtained a description of the tinnitus and the circumstances of its onset. It is important to not focus on the *sound* of the tinnitus. The purpose of any treatment is to help patients learn how to manage the *effects* of tinnitus—not to try to change its sound in any way.

Question 1: Does the loudness of your tinnitus seem to change for no apparent reason?

People may report the loudness of their tinnitus changes when exposed to certain sounds, eating certain foods, experiencing extreme stress or sleep deprivation, and taking new medications or changing dosages. Answering this question should not reflect these types of situations. The intent is to determine whether the loudness of the tinnitus changes *for no apparent reason*, and if so, how often. "For no apparent reason" means *spontaneous* changes in loudness—not caused by any known situation or event. Why is this important?

People often report that their tinnitus "spiked" in loudness and for no known reason. This increased loudness tends to get their attention and worsen any effects they are experiencing because of their tinnitus. Discussing these seemingly spontaneous increases in loudness is important so that they understand that such fluctuations are normal and no cause for alarm. At other times, they may be aware that their tinnitus becomes louder when they are stressed, sleep-deprived, or when they ingest certain foods or drugs. It's part of the education that people need to be informed about what it means when their tinnitus fluctuates and to be able to handle these changes without being unduly concerned.

Tinnitus may become more bothersome if the tinnitus becomes louder. Conversely, it may become less noticeable if it becomes softer. The main objective with PTM is to teach people how to *manage effects of tinnitus when it is bothersome*. It is therefore important to help them handle any spontaneous increases in its loudness that might make it more bothersome.

Question 2: Do sounds ever change the loudness of your tinnitus? (if "louder") What kinds of sounds make your tinnitus louder? When sound makes your tinnitus louder, how long does the change last?

People sometimes report that exposure to certain sounds increases the loudness of their tinnitus.[5,49] Dangerously loud sounds would be expected to have this effect. In chapter 5 it was explained that exposure to loud noise can damage the hair cells in the cochlea, causing or worsening hearing loss and/or tinnitus.[10,128]

If the patient responds "louder" to this question and checks that the effect is caused by "very loud sounds," such a response might be expected. These patients should be counseled about the need to protect their ears from dangerously loud sound.

The intent of the question, however, is to find out whether sounds at *non-damaging levels* cause an increase in tinnitus loudness. The effect may last minutes or hours, but the concern is whether it lasts to the next morning. Credit is given to Tinnitus Retraining Therapy (TRT) for raising this concern.[49] With TRT, these patients might be placed in a special category indicating successful treatment may be more challenging than usual.

Patients who experience prolonged tinnitus worsening due to non-damaging levels of sound should be advised to carry earplugs to be prepared for unavoidable situations that could expose them to sounds that make their tinnitus worse. The ideal might be custom-fit high-fidelity earplugs (also referred to as *musicians* earplugs), which reduce the level of sound evenly across the frequency range—they maintain the full spectrum of sound while making the sound safe for the ears. They require ear impressions made by an audiologist that are sent to a lab to make the custom earplugs.

People who experience prolonged worsening of tinnitus from sound may also require treatment for loudness hyperacusis, which is a heightened sensitivity to the loudness of sound.[92,93] When counseling patients about the use of earplugs, it's essential to caution them to *avoid overuse* of earplugs, which can increase their tinnitus and any sensitivity to sound.[181]

Question 3: How does your tinnitus affect your life (not including trouble hearing or understanding speech)?

This is a purposely open-ended question without any response choices listed. By being open-ended, it should prompt a response that reveals the most significant tinnitus-related concerns. People *just know* how tinnitus affects their life, and this question gives them the opportunity to express their biggest concerns *in their own words*. The response can be very revealing and will most likely indicate the primary complaint(s) that should be targeted by treatment. To ensure that the tinnitus is not being blamed for a hearing problem, the question is followed by "not including trouble hearing or understanding speech."

Question 4: Please describe everything you tried for your tinnitus prior to PTM. For each effort, what were you hoping would happen, and what actually did happen?

Following the question, a note to the clinician explains the main purpose of asking the question, which is to determine whether the person's efforts are focused on "making the tinnitus quieter." That would be a fruitless effort because nothing has been discovered to make tinnitus quieter, which would of course be a partial cure.

If the person has made repeated attempts to quiet the tinnitus, it is possible that each unsuccessful effort just added to the person's frustration. If this has been the person's pattern of help-seeking, then it should be restated that the goal of treatment with PTM (or any tinnitus treatment) is not to change the tinnitus in any way, but rather to *manage its effects*. This can be a difficult concept to convey to the person who has trouble accepting any treatment that will not make the tinnitus quieter.

Question 5: Please describe the sounds you have used to manage your reactions to tinnitus since starting PTM. For each sound you tried, what were you hoping would happen, and what actually did happen?

This question asks for the person's impressions regarding the use of therapeutic sound to reduce effects of tinnitus. Ideally, any Sound Plan Worksheets that were used by the person would be available to assist in answering the question. It is an opportunity to identify unrealistic expectations or misunderstandings regarding specific uses of sound, which would indicate the need to reinstruct the person to correct any confusion. It is especially helpful to point out any successes that have been noted. Even small successes will encourage continued efforts to discover what kinds of sounds can be helpful in different tinnitus-problem situations.

Question 6: If we decide to move ahead with one-on-one support, then we will be making plans for using sound to manage your reactions to tinnitus. It will be helpful to have a list of sound-producing devices that you have available to you. Which of the following devices do you own?

Sound therapy can involve any type of sound and any type of sound-producing device. This question lists common sound-producing devices and asks if any of these are available. If so, a series of questions ask for more detail (How many are available? Are any portable? If not portable, where is it located? How is it being used with respect to tinnitus?) The idea is to remind people not to overlook sounds and sound devices they already own that can be used for sound therapy. Creating this list can be helpful to create and modify Sound Plan Worksheets.

What About Hearing Aids?

At the Level 2 Audiology Evaluation, patients undergo a hearing aid assessment if the test results indicate hearing aids might be beneficial. Ideally, any patient who would benefit from hearing aids would receive and use them. This is not always the case, as seen by the low rates of hearing aid use by people with hearing loss.[182]

In chapter 3 it was mentioned that hearing aids can be considered a variation of sound therapy simply because they amplify sound in the environment.[1] There is considerable evidence that hearing aids can be beneficial for reducing effects of tinnitus regardless of the degree of hearing loss.[183-187]

Hearing aids can even help people who have normal hearing along with their bothersome tinnitus. Many audiologists are fitting hearing aids as treatment for tinnitus. There is scientific support for this practice.[188] Also, mild-gain hearing aids have been shown to be helpful to some people who have normal hearing sensitivity but difficulty understanding speech in a noisy background.[189,190]

> ...hearing aids can be beneficial for reducing effects of tinnitus regardless of the degree of hearing loss.

During the Level 4 Interdisciplinary Evaluation, the question of hearing aid use should be revisited. If the person already wears hearing aids, the aids should be evaluated to determine whether they are performing adequately to address the hearing loss. Since tinnitus is the main concern at Level 4, it is important to determine whether the hearing aids contain a built-in sound generator or have the capability of streaming sounds from a smartphone. If not, then different hearing aids should be considered that have those features. It is possible that a person's hearing aids already have these features but they have not yet been utilized.

In short, if the person is already wearing hearing aids, then the aids should be optimized for use as sound therapy devices for tinnitus. Hearing aids with additional tinnitus-treatment features greatly expand on the sound therapy capabilities of the devices. With PTM, all possibilities for delivering sound therapy are considered.

> With PTM, all possibilities for delivering sound therapy are considered.

If patients who reach Level 4 are *not* wearing hearing aids, then the audiologist should explain the potential benefits of using hearing aids. Amplification can be helpful to increase the level of ambient sound, which makes the tinnitus less noticeable. Built-in sound generators can be used to either partially or completely mask the tinnitus. Streaming features enable any sound to be accessed from the internet by a smartphone and presented directly to the ears.

Use of hearing aids or combination devices requires ongoing support from an audiologist, which would involve continued development and assessment of strategies for using sound most effectively.[82] Accordingly, the Sound Plan Worksheet (Fig. 9-4) should be reviewed and updated at every appointment.

Level 4 Evaluation by a Psychologist

Progressing through the different stepped-care levels of PTM ensures that any person who reaches Level 4 really does require an in-depth tinnitus evaluation.[82] These people are more likely to have psychological conditions or sleep disorders that would indicate the need for specialized services to evaluate and treat those conditions. Whereas *treatment* with CBT can be performed by any competent psychological health clinician, Level 4 specifically requires a psychologist (or psychiatrist) because they are qualified to *diagnose* mental health conditions and sleep disorders (as explained in the introduction to this chapter).

Evaluation by a psychologist involves testing for conditions that coexist with tinnitus.

Evaluation by a psychologist involves testing for conditions that coexist with tinnitus. "It is now agreed that the most common problems associated with tinnitus are sleep disturbance, emotional disturbance and concentration problems, as well as auditory perceptual disorders such as interference with hearing or increased sensitivity to noise (Hallam et al., 1988[191])"[192] (p. 93) *Auditory perceptual disorders* are addressed by audiologists. *Sleep disturbance, emotional disturbance, and concentration problems* are addressed indirectly by sound therapy and directly by psychological health providers during the Level 3 Skills Education sessions. At Level 4, psychologists evaluate patients mainly for sleep disturbance, emotional disturbance, and concentration problems.

Any psychologist would conduct the Level 4 evaluation somewhat differently. Many questionnaires can be used to evaluate and diagnose the different problems. The section below includes certain tests that would be appropriate, but many other tests are available that are not mentioned. The main intent here is to show how a psychologist might go about the Level 4 evaluation.

Sleep Disturbance

As mentioned in previous chapters, sleep problems (insomnia) are the most common effect of tinnitus.[135,136] They also may be the most *significant* complaint.[192] Sleep disturbance can involve difficulty falling asleep, difficulty returning to sleep after waking, and waking up early in the morning and not being able to get back to sleep. These difficulties have been described as "sleep being light, broken, or restless, and not being restorative or refreshing. Complaints about associated daytime problems

> ...sleep problems (insomnia) are the most common effect of tinnitus.

such as tiredness or sleepiness, mood disturbance, and poor performance are also common."[193] (pp. 83-84)

Diagnosing a sleep disturbance may be primarily a matter of clinical judgment by the psychologist.[193] Making the diagnosis, however, can be based on certain criteria: (1) it takes the person at least 30 minutes to either fall asleep or get back to sleep after waking; (2) the total time awake during the night when trying to sleep is 45 minutes or more; (3) the total amount of sleep is less than six hours on a given night; and (4) any of these first three problems occurs three or more times per week. These are not rigid criteria, but they recognize the critical need for sleep *quality* as well as the *quantity* of sleep. A sleep diary completed nightly may be the best means of assessing a sleep disorder.[194]

Patients attending the Level 2 Audiology Evaluation are asked, "Do you have trouble sleeping?" If so, the seven-item Insomnia Severity Index (ISI) is available to evaluate the degree to which insomnia is a problem.[137] A score of at least 10 indicates a significant problem with insomnia. If sleep continues to be a problem for the person at Level 4, then the ISI may be used by the psychologist.

The Epworth Sleepiness Scale (ESS) is widely used to assess a person's general level of daytime sleepiness.[195,196] A score of 10 or more suggests that the person is not getting adequate sleep. Sleep quality can also be assessed with the Pittsburgh Sleep Quality Index (PSQI).[197] An advantage of the PSQI is that it assesses sleep quality with respect to seven different aspects of sleep.[194] Each aspect can be scored separately, and all seven provide a global PSQI score.

Insomnia does not normally necessitate referral to a sleep clinic unless there are also symptoms of sleep-disordered breathing (sleep apnea—snoring, morning headaches, etc.), rapid eye movement (REM) behavior disorder (acting out a dream, often by punching, kicking, and thrashing), or narcolepsy (excessive daytime sleepiness).[82,198-200] These symptoms, which usually are not related to tinnitus, can indicate a serious medical condition (for example, severe sleep apnea increases the risk for heart attack and stroke) that may require medical treatment.[201]

Anxiety and Depression

Anxiety and depression are commonly reported conditions experienced by tinnitus clinic patients.[105,202] It is always a question whether these psychological conditions affect how tinnitus is experienced, or if tinnitus causes or worsens anxiety and/or depression. Regardless, symptoms of anxiety and depression need to be evaluated by the psychologist. Screening for both can be done using the Hospital Anxiety and Depression Scale (HADS).[203] More comprehensive measures of anxiety and depression are available.[204,205]

Trauma-Related Tinnitus

Tinnitus often develops after traumatic injuries—especially those affecting the ear.[206,207] Such trauma can include sudden exposure to excessively loud noise, brain injuries, neck injuries, and emotional trauma. A study of over 1,600 tinnitus patients revealed clear differences between those with trauma versus those without trauma preceding their tinnitus onset.[24] Those with trauma, especially whiplash or head trauma, were more impacted than those without trauma. It therefore appears that these two groups represent different subtypes of patients with tinnitus.

Patients should be systematically evaluated by the psychologist to determine whether they have trauma-related tinnitus. If so, symptoms of post-traumatic stress disorder (PTSD) should be assessed[23,25] to tailor the treatment approach to the individual. "The consequences of trauma may produce a number of powerful symptoms that endure long after the trauma's conclusion. When tinnitus and trauma are intertwined in the emotional state and life of the patient, any efforts at symptom management will be complicated and challenging due to the variety of powerful influences."[23] (p. 9)

Other Psychological Conditions

In addition to what has been covered, many other evaluations can be performed by a psychologist. Any number of non-auditory problems can be involved, and psychologists are trained in diagnosing these various conditions.[192] In some cases the tinnitus is the primary source of the problem. In other cases, these conditions are independent of the tinnitus.

"The different factors within the tinnitus complaint offer different therapeutic goals. . . . There is, therefore, a very real value in identifying the moderating factors which lead some people to suffer more than others. A profile of vulnerability, involving personality factors, general anxiety and crucial life stress, was identified by Erlandsson (2000).[136]

These factors, together with others such as coping style, family relationships, general health and possibly environment, may all play some part in determining the overall effect that tinnitus has on a person's life."[192] (p. 111)

Level 5 Individualized Support Needed?

After the audiologist and psychologist have completed the Level 4 evaluation, a decision needs to be made whether further services are needed. If so, then the person would be advised to receive Level 5 Individualized Support (described in the next chapter). This decision is made by the psychologist, audiologist, and patient communicating with one another about the results of the evaluation. The clinicians may make recommendations, but the patient makes the final decision.

In general, the following conditions should be met before a person is scheduled to receive Level 5 services:

> The clinicians may make recommendations, but the patient makes the final decision.

- Levels 1 through 4 of PTM have been insufficient in resolving the tinnitus-related effects.
- The Level 4 evaluation indicates the need for further treatment.
- The person is fully informed about options available for Level 5 treatment.

- The person is motivated and capable of participating in the proposed treatment.

If all these conditions are met, then the person progresses to receive Level 5 Individualized Support.

CHAPTER 13

PTM Level 5 Individualized Support

Level 5 is unstructured and flexible to allow any number of treatment approaches to be offered to the patient who reaches this stage of PTM. In this chapter we discuss some of the different approaches to treatment that would be options for Level 5. Patients reaching this level have been fully evaluated by a psychologist and an audiologist (Level 4), and it should be evident what issues they are dealing with that require intervention.

Options for Level 5 Treatment

One approach is to continue with the treatment that was provided in Level 3 Skills Education. For an individual patient, it's possible that the strategies taught during Level 3 might have been appropriate, but for some reason they were not successful (the reason should be made clear during the Level 4 evaluation). The skills taught during the Level 3 sessions do not necessarily resonate with everyone; further instruction may be needed so that the patient fully grasps the purpose for learning these skills and how to implement them in daily life.

The audiologist can meet with the patient one-on-one to optimize the use of sound to treat the effects of tinnitus in any situation when tinnitus is bothersome. The audiology counseling information is essentially the same as what was covered during the Level 3 sessions. The more informal structure of the Level 5 counseling allows for slower-paced and more personalized interaction than can be provided in Level 3. A flip-chart counseling book is available to guide the counseling—both for the audiologist and the patient.[98] The psychologist (or other psychological health provider) can review the CBT strategies that were taught in Level 3 and possibly teach new CBT strategies. If both the psychologist and audiologist provide Level 5 services, they should remain in regular contact to discuss the patient's progress.

The psychologist may have expertise in third wave CBT, which includes mindfulness-based approaches (mindfulness-based stress reduction and acceptance and commitment therapy). Third wave approaches to CBT are becoming increasingly popular as treatment for many health conditions, including tinnitus.[51,70,71] Having already learned the basic CBT skills taught during Level 3, patients have the foundation to learn the third wave approach to CBT.

It also may be that a person has difficulty attending in-person sessions. Providing tinnitus counseling via telehealth is an option for any patient who has difficulty attending in-person sessions for any reason. PTM has been shown effective for treating tinnitus via telephone (Tele-PTM).[95,208] Tele-PTM would of course be an option for Level 5 and could include remote counseling from both the audiologist and the psychologist (or other psychological health provider). Third wave CBT could be provided via telehealth.

Internet-based CBT has been shown to be effective for many different health conditions, including conditions that may coexist with bothersome tinnitus.[209] A number of trials have been conducted using internet-based CBT as treatment for tinnitus with positive results.[176,210]

It may be determined that the person would likely benefit from a different form of therapy. If that's the case, then it opens up a huge array of different treatments to choose from. We'll start with those I mentioned in chapter 3 as being "established" treatments, including Tinnitus Retraining Therapy and Tinnitus Activities Treatment. Tinnitus Retraining Therapy involves extensive counseling that is unique and highly structured and can be provided by an audiologist.[5,49] Tinnitus Activities Treatment also offers a unique approach to counseling.[73,74,78]

Books Describing Treatments for Tinnitus

It is not possible in this chapter to review all of the various treatments that might be available to patients in Level 5. Books are available that describe a variety of treatments for tinnitus. For example, Tyler and Perreau edited a scholarly book that covers sensory meditation and mindfulness, smartphone apps, various counseling and sound therapy approaches, tinnitus-related insomnia, hearing aids, relaxation and distraction techniques (guided imagery, progressive muscle relaxation, biofeedback, music therapy, art therapy, exercise), and emerging treatments (transcranial magnetic stimulation, vagus nerve stimulation).[211]

Another scholarly book I would recommend was edited by Deshpande and Hall.[212] That book covers at-home tinnitus therapy options, hearing aids, audiologist-delivered CBT, Tele-PTM, dietary supplements, cannabis-derived products, essential oils, and complementary and alternative approaches.

More excellent books are available.[192,213,214] It should be noted, however, that the books I've mentioned are intended for professionals. That does not mean the lay reader could not benefit from them. A number of books are written specifically for the consumer, all of which can be helpful in self-learning about different approaches to tinnitus treatment.[5,62,180,215]

Suggestions for Deciding on Level 5 Treatment

With all the treatments for tinnitus that are available, it can be a daunting task to decide which to use. My advice would be to, first, avoid making a decision based on what you might find on the internet, which offers a plethora of books and dietary supplements. The books I've cited

...avoid making a decision based on what you might find on the internet...

have good information, but a great many books are not particularly helpful. No dietary supplement has been shown to be effective for treating tinnitus, in spite of their popularity. A well-balanced review of dietary supplements, vitamins, essential oils, and cannabidiol (CBD) oils advertised for tinnitus relief is available.[216]

My second piece of advice would be to try methods that are either free or low cost and that cannot cause any harm. These methods would include apps, of which there are many. Some of these apps provide different options for sound therapy

> ...try methods that are either free or low cost and that cannot cause any harm.

and some offer counseling advice, including CBT. As already mentioned, numerous online programs offer CBT or other forms of counseling. Whether an app or an online therapy program, the user needs to be motivated to follow through with the program. The self-help books I cited above can also be beneficial.[5,62,180,215]

A person may rule out free or low-cost options. Different options might have been tried without success. Or the person, for whatever reason, is not motivated to make the effort to try them. Therapy with one of the established methods (chapter 3) would be the next step, although those methods are only offered by a limited number of clinicians. If none of these is possible, then different commercial methods might be considered. These methods, however, can be costly and may not have the same level of evidence as the more established methods. That does not mean they can't be effective. The concern is that a person might pay a lot of money for some method that has not been shown to be any more effective than a placebo. I have addressed this concern in chapter 3.

The scientific evidence (systematic reviews and clinical practice guidelines) favors CBT for bothersome tinnitus. It's important to know, however, that evidence-based practice consists of more than just scientific evidence. Scientific evidence is one of three essential components, the other two being the expertise of the clinician and the preferences of the person receiving the treatment.[217] It can be thought of as a three-legged stool—all three legs are necessary or the stool doesn't work. The three legs are best research evidence, clinical expertise, and patient preferences.

Summary

Ultimately, Level 5 is all about finding a method of treatment that will help the patient establish a quality of life that is mostly unaffected by the tinnitus. Patients who reach Level 5 have undergone multiple levels of assessment and treatment that provide reasonable assurance that individualized clinical attention is needed. They may be frustrated and discouraged, and compassionate care is essential. Any treatment provided in Level 5 should be continued for as long as necessary.

CHAPTER 14

Telehealth Progressive Tinnitus Management (Tele-PTM)

The ability to provide clinical services remotely (via *telehealth*) has greatly expanded opportunities for people to receive tinnitus services.[218] Tele-PTM is the telehealth version of PTM. Not only has PTM received substantial research but Tele-PTM has also. The method was developed and pilot-tested with good results.[208] Following the pilot study, the method was refined and a randomized controlled trial with 209 participants was completed.[95] Both of these studies are briefly described in appendix A. Tele-PTM is not just a concept but a well-researched method of providing tinnitus counseling to people regardless of their geographic location.

Overview of Tele-PTM

The essence of Tele-PTM is that it provides PTM Levels 3, 4, and 5 services remotely.[218] Tele-PTM can take over with a patient who has been properly referred and evaluated but does not have access to high-quality tinnitus treatment. The Level 2 Audiology Evaluation must be done in person by an audiologist. Fortunately, audiologists are in every town and all of them have knowledge about tinnitus. As described in chapter 6, the Level 2 evaluation involves testing that an audiologist would normally do, plus completing the Tinnitus and Hearing Survey.[91] The Level 2 test results would need to be provided to the Tele-PTM clinician who does the screening to determine whether it is appropriate for the person to receive the remote treatment. If the Tinnitus and Hearing Survey was not completed, it is always administered by the Tele-PTM screening clinician as part of the evaluation for the Tele-PTM program.

Any candidate for Tele-PTM should have hearing aids if needed for hearing loss. The hearing aids should be optimized for tinnitus management, including sound generators and/or streaming capability if possible. Because of the known benefits of hearing aids for reducing effects of tinnitus,[185,219-221] it would be pointless to provide tinnitus counseling if hearing aids might address the concerns. More is said about the use of hearing aids as treatment for tinnitus throughout this book and in appendix A.

Tele-PTM Screening

A screening interview needs to first take place between the individual and a Tele-PTM clinician. Ideally, the clinician would be a psychologist who can do psychological screening to ensure the Tele-PTM counseling will be appropriate for the individual.

Screening determines whether the person has received an audiology evaluation and hearing aids if needed. The Tinnitus and Hearing Survey ensures that the person is not blaming the tinnitus for any hearing problems. If necessary, the Tinnitus Screener can be used if there is any question whether the person has tinnitus or just "ear noise" (see chapter 2).[7,8] The Tinnitus Functional Index (or another tinnitus questionnaire) can be administered to better understand the tinnitus-related concerns.[20]

Tele-PTM Procedures

After enrollment, the Tele-PTM procedures are usually straightforward. Prior to the counseling, a medical history is conducted and the Tinnitus Functional Index (TFI) is administered as a baseline for outcome assessment (the medical history and TFI are described, respectively, in chapters 6 and 7).

The Level 3 counseling is then performed in the same manner as for in-person counseling. That includes two sessions of sound therapy by the audiologist (described in chapter 9) and three sessions of CBT by the psychologist (described in chapter 10). Following the counseling, the One-Week Post-Treatment Survey (appendix B) and Six-Week Post-Treatment Interview (appendix C) are administered. Administering each of these post-treatment instruments is described in chapter 11.

Finally, the Tinnitus Functional Index is administered along with determining whether the patient believes there has been improvement (explained in chapter 7). The two questions in Figure 7-1 (Impression of Change-in-Tinnitus-Impact Questions) are used along with the TFI. These measures usually agree, but occasionally they do not. The main question is whether treatment was considered successful by the patient. If so, then treatment is complete.

If all of this has been done and the patient is not satisfied, then further evaluation may be necessary to attempt to determine why treatment was not successful. The evaluation would be comparable to what is described in chapter 12 for the PTM Level 4 Interdisciplinary Evaluation. If further therapy is required, then other treatment approaches can be considered. Many different options for treatment are mentioned in chapter 13.

As for PTM Level 5, Tele-PTM treatment can continue for as long as necessary to meet the person's needs. The treatment can be repeated or revised, or it can shift to another method completely. Other methods would typically include acceptance and commitment therapy, mindfulness training, Tinnitus Retraining Therapy, or Tinnitus Activities Treatment.

> ...Tele-PTM treatment can continue for as long as necessary to meet the person's needs.

Some of these methods can be conducted online, such as internet-based CBT.[209]

There are also hundreds of sound therapy apps that can be used. Many are either free or very inexpensive. They often contain an extensive number of sounds along with the ability to combine and/or modify the sounds. Also available are a variety of relaxation app, podcasts, and audiobooks. The internet provides many options for treating tinnitus.

Summary

Tele-PTM can meet the needs of many people who have bothersome tinnitus but do not have access to competent tinnitus services. People can be located anywhere and complete the procedures described in this chapter. Tele-PTM practically eliminates the concern that these needed services are inaccessible. There may be issues related to providing healthcare services across state boundaries or borders between countries. Fortunately, the sessions can be considered "educational." This is a licensing question that needs to be addressed on a per-state or per-country basis.

PART 5

Wrap-Up

CHAPTER 15

Summary, Suggestions, and Resources

Summary

The development of PTM is the result of many years of research conducted by a team of dedicated individuals. Appendix A describes the sequence of activities that led to PTM and then to Tele-PTM. The team included clinicians who practiced the procedures in their clinics. We had the great fortune of combining results from our research studies with experiences of clinicians in the field. The VA healthcare system made this research possible because it is an integrated network of hospitals and clinics.

An overview of PTM is provided in chapter 4. It is therefore not necessary to repeat the overview here. Key features of PTM are that it is a stepped-care program and relies on both audiologists and psychological health providers as the primary clinicians who perform the procedures. Patients are referred to an ear-specialist physician if they have symptoms of secondary tinnitus ("sound vibrations in the head"). Otherwise, audiologists can do the basic assessment (Level 2), and audiologists and psychological health providers each have a role in the treatment.

Suggestions to Optimize Success with PTM

As already mentioned, it is recommended that people with tinnitus have their hearing tested by an audiologist because of the likelihood they also have hearing loss. Regardless of any other symptoms a person experiences, a hearing evaluation is essential. Audiologists are trained to know if referral out to another provider is needed. The question is always, "Does the person need treatment to address tinnitus-specific problems?" That question is usually answered if the person completes the Tinnitus and Hearing Survey during the hearing evaluation appointment.

Suggestion #1: Make sure to complete the Tinnitus and Hearing Survey during your audiology appointment and discuss the results with your audiologist.

The Level 2 Audiology Evaluation may result in a decision that treatment is needed. It may be difficult, however, to make an *informed* decision about treatment without being educated about the basics of tinnitus—how and why it becomes a problem and what realistically can be done about it. For this reason, anyone considering treatment should be provided with the opportunity to receive this basic education by attending a class, watching a video, or receiving written information.

Suggestion #2: Only agree to receive tinnitus-specific treatment if you have been fully educated about how and why tinnitus becomes a problem and what realistically can be done about it.

Those who complete the audiology evaluation and receive the basic tinnitus education may decide that further tinnitus services are not needed. If so, then their tinnitus care is complete. If treatment is needed, then they will plan to receive Level 3 Skills Education. Level 3 involves five sessions—two with an audiologist and three with a psychological health provider. The intent of these sessions is to learn self-care skills to know what to do whenever tinnitus is bothersome. Learning these skills takes motivation and practice to identify strategies that are helpful. These strategies are often different for different situations when tinnitus is bothersome. Without putting in the effort to practice the skills, just learning about them will have minimal benefit.

Suggestion #3: Plan to receive the Level 3 treatment only if you are motivated to learn the skills and to practice them on a regular basis.

Completing Level 3 is successful for most people. That means any problems they were having with tinnitus have been sufficiently reduced such that treatment is no longer necessary.

Suggestion #4: After Level 3 treatment is received, it is essential to complete the follow-up evaluations (One-Week Post-Treatment Survey and Six-Week Post-Treatment Interview—appendixes B and C, respectively) to ensure that no further tinnitus services are needed or wanted.

> Very few people
> require services
> beyond Level 3.

Very few people require services beyond Level 3. If they do, then a comprehensive evaluation is conducted at the Level 4 Interdisciplinary Evaluation, which requires about an hour with an audiologist and an hour with a psychologist. These evaluations are designed to determine why services to this point have not been sufficient in resolving the tinnitus problem. Undergoing these evaluations requires patients to be completely open about why tinnitus might be so bothersome. They may have to answer some uncomfortable questions, especially by the psychologist about any possible mental health concerns.

Suggestion #5: If you are receiving the Level 4 evaluation, it is essential to be completely transparent about any possible causes for the tinnitus distress, including the possibility of psychological health issues.

If the Level 4 evaluation determines that Level 5 Individualized Support is needed, a range of treatment options requires decisions to determine what form of treatment might be most helpful. It is important at this stage to be aware of all the options and to choose on the basis of what would realistically be expected to resolve the effects of tinnitus. It might be tempting to pay for an expensive commercial product or service, but low-cost options should be considered before spending a lot of money on treatment. There is no proof that any one method works better than any other, and that includes everything from free apps to products costing thousands of dollars.

Suggestion #6: Make wise and informed decisions about what treatment might be best for long-term care for tinnitus, with special consideration of any costs involved.

Following these suggestions should help in getting the best possible results from PTM. Treatment is a process of learning what to do in every situation when tinnitus is a problem. Treatment is not a one-size-fits-all approach, so different situations may require different

> Treatment is a process of learning what to do in every situation when tinnitus is a problem.

strategies. The main goal with PTM is to learn situation-specific strategies, which are ultimately tools to enable the person to live a normal life in spite of the ongoing presence of tinnitus.

PTM Resources

The book you are reading now is the best PTM resource I can offer. Throughout the book I have cited references that support different claims and statements. Any of those references can be useful resources. The PTM-specific references are the most relevant resources to what is contained in this book.[65,82,83,94-96,98,100,101,208,222-228]

The development of PTM took place primarily at the Veterans Affairs (VA) National Center for Rehabilitative Auditory Research (NCRAR) in Portland, Oregon. The NCRAR has a website, and on the tinnitus page a series of links are provided to access the different materials that have been mentioned throughout this book (https://www.ncrar.research.va.gov/Tinnitus/Index.asp).

I have my own website, and I am always willing to provide any needed PTM materials or to show where they may be obtained. (https://www.earsgonewrong.org). The NCRAR website is the best resource for these materials.

Parting Words

As we come to a close, may I just say what a pleasure it has been to write this book and to make it available to people who are struggling with tinnitus and to the clinicians who are dedicated to providing them with the needed clinical services. I am available to answer questions about tinnitus, and I invite you to contact me through my website.

PART 6

Appendixes

APPENDIX A

Research Evidence for Progressive Tinnitus Management

The National Center for Rehabilitative Auditory Research (NCRAR) was established in 1997 at the Portland Veterans Affairs Medical Center (PVAMC) in Portland, Oregon. Tinnitus research at the NCRAR traces back to my being hired as a research audiologist at the PVAMC in 1987. Because I wanted to start my own research program, I returned to school at Oregon Health & Science University (OHSU) in 1988 to earn a doctorate, which I completed in 1994. For those six years I worked part-time at the PVAMC and my doctoral training lab was the Oregon Hearing Research Center (OHRC), which is the research arm of the Department of Otolaryngology-Head & Neck Surgery at OHSU. At the time, the OHRC housed the OHSU Tinnitus Clinic, which was directed by Dr. Jack Vernon.[1] Dr. Vernon is well known for pioneering tinnitus research and developing the masking technique for tinnitus treatment.[40]

At the OHRC, Dr. Mary Meikle, another tinnitus pioneer, was my research adviser. Under her mentorship, I completed two research projects to earn a PhD. Both projects focused on different aspects of measuring tinnitus.[2,3] Completing these projects set the stage for me to further pursue tinnitus research, resulting in my first funded research grant in 1995. Tinnitus research was thus already underway at the PVAMC when the NCRAR was first established in 1997. Working with various research staff, I conducted tinnitus research continually from 1995 to 2022. A summary of my tinnitus research projects, along with other tinnitus research conducted at the NCRAR, was recently published.[229] Only the clinical research pertinent to PTM is reviewed in this appendix.

We first introduced the concept of a stepped-care method of tinnitus management in 2005.[83] In 2006 we received funding to develop and pilot-test PTM. About two years were spent developing the program, followed by a pilot trial of the method. We learned a great deal from this pilot study and PTM was modified accordingly, resulting in the protocol that was used in the studies described below.[82,97,98] Because the strongest research evidence is normally obtained by conducting randomized controlled trials (RCTs), I will just review the different RCTs that have been conducted for PTM.

PTM Multisite RCT

This RCT was conducted at two VA hospitals—one in Memphis, Tennessee, and the other in West Haven, Connecticut.[96]

At each site, 150 military Veterans were enrolled into the study (300 participants total) and randomized to either receive PTM Level 3 Skills Education (described in chapters 8, 9, and 10) or be placed on a six-month wait list (no treatment for six months). The Level 3 Skills Education involved two sessions of sound therapy instruction from an audiologist and three sessions of learning CBT coping skills from a psychologist.

Results of this RCT showed statistically significant improvement for the PTM group for all outcome measures, including the Tinnitus Functional Index (TFI). The improvement was statistically significantly better for the PTM group versus the wait-list group. These differences were consistent across the two study sites.

It is noteworthy that this was considered a *clinically embedded* study, meaning study participants were actual patients in clinics rather than having been recruited to participate in a study conducted in a laboratory. Such a study has advantages and disadvantages. The main advantage is that participants truly represented patients who seek routine care for their tinnitus. Another advantage is that the researchers learn about barriers (hindrances) and facilitators (enablers) to conducting the procedures in clinics.

A disadvantage of a clinically embedded study is that all patients are considered qualified candidates to participate in the study. This meant that some of the participants did not have tinnitus that was bothersome enough to warrant receiving the treatment that was offered. Evidence of that concern was the high number of patients who signed up for the treatment but then either did not show up or did not attend all the sessions. In spite of these concerns, PTM

THE PROGRESSIVE TINNITUS MANAGEMENT BOOK

was seen to be beneficial for reducing the effects of tinnitus for patients who were interested in attending the Level 3 sessions. These results compared favorably to RCTs that evaluated the use of CBT for tinnitus.

Tele-PTM

PTM Level 3 Skills Education was adapted to create an individualized, telephone-based treatment (Tele-PTM) that was administered to Veterans and non-Veterans located throughout the United States. A major purpose was to develop and validate tinnitus treatment for Veterans who had experienced a traumatic brain injury (TBI) and also had bothersome tinnitus. The study therefore targeted such individuals for enrollment, but many participants had bothersome tinnitus without a history of TBI.

We first developed and pilot-tested Tele-PTM.[208] All three groups in this pilot study had bothersome tinnitus. Fifteen had experienced a mild TBI, nine a moderate to severe TBI, and twelve had no history of a TBI. They all received the Level 3 counseling, which involved six sessions over six months with an audiologist and a psychologist. All groups showed similar improvement in their tinnitus questionnaire scores.

Following up on the pilot study, the Tele-PTM protocol was slightly modified, and an RCT was completed with 205 participants.[95] Recruitment took place nationwide at mostly VA and military hospitals. Participants were randomized to either receive the PTM Level 3 Skills Education or be placed on a six-month wait list. Those receiving treatment had five telephone counseling appointments—three with a psychologist (teaching CBT) and two with an audiologist (teaching sound therapy).

Results of this study showed convincingly that participants receiving remote treatment with PTM Level 3 Skills Education had statistically significantly better outcomes than the wait-list controls. These results provide strong support for the use of Tele-PTM with individuals who have bothersome tinnitus, regardless of whether they have experienced a TBI.

Hearing Aids for Tinnitus Management

Both of the previous RCTs evaluated PTM Level 3 Skills Education. We also conducted two RCTs that evaluated PTM Level 2 Audiology Evaluation for outcomes of individuals who had bothersome tinnitus and started using hearing aids. Hearing aids have long been reported to provide benefit for reducing effects of tinnitus.[185,219-221]

Many hearing aids incorporate built-in sound generators to provide relief from tinnitus. It was unknown if these *combination instruments* were more effective than hearing aids alone for tinnitus management. To address this question we conducted a small RCT.[186] Thirty individuals who had bothersome tinnitus and were qualified to use hearing aids were enrolled. Each participant was randomized to wear either hearing aids or combination instruments (all devices supplied by Starkey Hearing Technologies) for three months. Both groups showed statistically significant improvement based on reductions in TFI scores. The improvement was not statistically significant between groups, suggesting that both hearing aids and combination instruments are approximately equally effective in managing effects of tinnitus.

We conducted another RCT to evaluate three different types of ear-level devices to provide relief from tinnitus: conventional hearing aids, combination instruments, and extended-wear, deep-fit hearing aids (Lyric) (all devices supplied by Phonak, LLC).[187] For this study, 55 individuals who had bothersome tinnitus and were qualified to use hearing aids were randomized to use one of these three types of devices (in each ear) for four months. Almost all of the participants showed statistically significant improvement in tinnitus symptoms based on the TFI scores. As for the previous study, there were no statistically significant differences between the three groups.

Participants in both the Starkey and Phonak studies generally had significant reductions in the effects of tinnitus. There was, however, no evidence that any one of the devices tested provided greater relief from tinnitus than another.

Summary and Conclusion

The main treatment level for PTM is Level 3 Skills Education. That level is treatment only, and we completed two RCTs that focused on evaluating outcomes of the Level 3 treatment. One was an RCT that was a clinically embedded study conducted at two sites with 300 participants.[96] The other was a telephone-based study with 205 participants located around the United States.[95] Both of these studies showed benefit that was statistically significant for the use of the Level 3 treatment.

PTM Level 2 Audiology Evaluation involves assessment of patients, but hearing aids can also be dispensed at Level 2. Hearing aids are used as amplification to treat hearing loss. They have been shown, however, to also be beneficial for reducing effects of tinnitus.[185,219-221] Combination instruments are hearing aids with built-in sound generators. We conducted two RCTs to compare hearing aids with combination instruments.[186,187] The second RCT also used a group of participants who wore deep-fit, extended-wear hearing aids (Lyric).[187] All of these devices tested showed significant benefit for reducing effects of tinnitus, although no significant differences were seen between any of the devices.

These studies support the contention that PTM provides treatment that is effective at both Level 2 Audiology Evaluation and Level 3 Skills Education. The methodology is based on many years of research that led to PTM and Tele-PTM. The method is being used in many clinics, and one clinic has reported positive outcome data for both 5-year and 10-year follow-ups with patients who attended Level 3 group sessions.[100,101] Numerous other studies have evaluated different aspects of PTM.[222,226-228]

APPENDIX B

One-Week Post-Treatment Survey

1. Have you been **using sound** to manage your reactions to tinnitus?

   YES

   If yes, how often?

   ☐ Very often
   ☐ Often
   ☐ Sometimes
   ☐ Rarely

   NO

   If no, why not?

   ☐ I don't need to do this
   ☐ It's not worth the trouble
   ☐ I don't know what to do
   ☐ I don't think it helps
   ☐ I don't like to do this
   ☐ Other:_____

2. Have you been **practicing relaxation techniques** (deep breathing and/or imagery) to manage your reactions to tinnitus?

YES   **NO**

If yes, how often?   **If no**, why not?

☐ Very often   ☐ I don't need to do this
☐ Often   ☐ It's not worth the trouble
☐ Sometimes   ☐ I don't know what to do
☐ Rarely   ☐ I don't think it helps
                      ☐ I don't like to do this
                      ☐ Other:_____

3. Have you been **planning more pleasant activities** to help manage your reactions to tinnitus?

YES   **NO**

If yes, how often?   **If no**, why not?

☐ Very often   ☐ I don't need to do this
☐ Often   ☐ It's not worth the trouble
☐ Sometimes   ☐ I don't know what to do
☐ Rarely   ☐ I don't think it helps
                      ☐ I don't like to do this
                      ☐ Other:_____

4. Have you been working on **changing your thoughts about tinnitus** to help you feel better?

   YES   **NO**

   If yes, how often?   **If no,** why not?

   ☐ Very often   ☐ I don't need to do this
   ☐ Often   ☐ It's not worth the trouble
   ☐ Sometimes   ☐ I don't know what to do
   ☐ Rarely   ☐ I don't think it helps
                                       ☐ I don't like to do this
                                       ☐ Other:_____

5. Compared to how I felt before the Level 3 sessions, **I now feel**:
   ☐ **A lot more in control** of my reactions to tinnitus
   ☐ **Somewhat more in control** of my reactions to tinnitus
   ☐ **A little more in control** of my reactions to tinnitus
   ☐ **The same (no change in control** of my reactions to tinnitus)

6. Compared to before the Level 3 sessions, my ability to **cope** with tinnitus is now:

A lot worse	Somewhat worse	A little worse	The same	A little better	Somewhat better	A lot better
☐	☐	☐	☐	☐	☐	☐

7. Compared to before the Level 3 sessions, my **quality of life** is now:

A lot worse	Somewhat worse	A little worse	The same	A little better	Somewhat better	A lot better
☐	☐	☐	☐	☐	☐	☐

8. Compared to before the Level 3 sessions, my tinnitus now **bothers me**:

A lot worse	Somewhat worse	A little worse	The same	A little better	Somewhat better	A lot better
☐	☐	☐	☐	☐	☐	☐

9. Would you **recommend the Level 3 Skills Education sessions** to someone else who has bothersome tinnitus?

 YES   NO

 If "no," please explain:_____

 _____

10. Please **describe your overall experience** learning how to manage your reactions to tinnitus.

 _____

 _____

 _____

APPENDIX C

Six-Week Post-Treatment Interview

The questions below are provided as a framework for guiding a conversation about how the patient has been doing since the PTM Level 3 Skills Education sessions. No specific criteria are provided to guide decision-making at the end of the interview. The clinician and patient discuss general progress and together make a decision about what to do next.

1. **Since the treatment, what have you been doing to manage how tinnitus affects your life?**

   _____

   _____

Use of sound?

_____

_____

Relaxation techniques?

_____

_____

Planning pleasant activities?

_____

_____

Changing thoughts?

_____

_____

Other comments?

_____

_____

2. **What has been <u>most</u> helpful for you?**

_____

_____

3. **What has been <u>least</u> helpful for yo u?**

_____

_____

4. **Overall, <u>how satisfied</u> are you with how you are doing with your tinnitus?**

_____

_____

Below are five options for how to proceed. Below each option is a description of who might be interested in that option. However, the decision for how to proceed is up to the judgment and desires of both clinician and patient (even in cases when the decision does not match the descriptors well).

- **No further intervention**
  - ▶ Reasonably satisfied with how well tinnitus is managed
  - ▶ Does not desire further intervention

- **If applicable, activate sound generator portion of ear-level combination instrument(s) with no further intervention**
  - ▶ Reasonably well satisfied with how well tinnitus is managed
  - ▶ Using skills learned from Level 3
  - ▶ Likely to benefit from addition of sound generator portion of ear-level device

- **Attend all sessions again**
  - ▶ Would like to review the content from all sessions
  - ▶ Would like to use the group interactions to provide motivation to carry through with using the techniques taught during all sessions

- **Attend some sessions again**
  - ▸ Would like to review content from certain sessions, but not all sessions
  - ▸ (If the session involved a group of patients) Would like to use group interactions to provide motivation to carry through with using some of the skills

- **Watch videos that provide content from the sessions**
  - ▸ Would like to review the content from the sessions, but does not wish to engage in group interactions again, or would prefer to review content without being required to return to the clinic

- **Level 4 Interdisciplinary Evaluation**
  - ▸ Desires further intervention, but repeating the sessions is undesirable and/or deemed unlikely to be helpful

PTM Level 4 Interdisciplinary Evaluation: Tinnitus Interview

This interview is intended to be completed immediately after completing the Tinnitus Functional Index and the Tinnitus and Hearing Survey and thoroughly discussing the results. (Please note this interview does not cover tinnitus-specific information that was covered as part of the case history that was done at the Level 2 Audiology Evaluation.)

1. Does the loudness of your tinnitus change *on its own*?
    - ☐ **No → Go to #2**
    - ☐ **Yes → How often does it change?**
        - ☐ **Never**
        - ☐ **Several times per month**
        - ☐ **Several times per week**
        - ☐ **Several times per day**
        - ☐ **Several times per hour**

2. Do sounds ever change the loudness of your tinnitus?
   - ☐ **No effect → Go to #3**
   - ☐ **Softer → Go to #3**
   - ☐ **Louder**

   (if "louder") **What kinds of sounds make your tinnitus louder? (check all categories that apply; circle any sounds that are identified as a problem; write in any additional sounds that are not mentioned)**

   - ☐ <u>Very loud sounds/activities</u> that would be expected to make the tinnitus louder (firing a gun, attending a concert, using power tools, _____)
     (***Clinician:*** *If this is the only response from the patient, then exacerbation of tinnitus by sound would be considered a normal effect.*)

   - ☐ <u>Higher-pitched sounds</u> (squeals, squeaks, beeps, whistles, rings, _____)

   - ☐ <u>Lower-pitched sounds</u> (bass from radio, _____)

   - ☐ <u>Traffic (warning) sounds</u> (emergency vehicle sirens, car horns, backup beeper on truck/van, _____)

   - ☐ <u>Traffic (background) sounds</u> (road noise, road construction, diesel engines, garbage trucks, _____)

   - ☐ <u>Sudden impact sounds</u> (door slam, car backfiring, objects dropping on floor, dishes clattering, _____)

☐ <u>Voices</u> (television, radio, movies, children's voices, dog barking, _____)

☐ <u>Other</u> (describe) _____

When sound makes your tinnitus louder, how long does the change last?

☐ 1–2	☐ **Second(s)**
☐ 3–4	☐ **Minute(s)**
☐ 5–10	☐ **Hour(s)**
☐ **more than 10**	☐ **Day(s)**

3. How does your tinnitus affect your life (not including trouble hearing or understanding speech)?_____
_____

4. Please describe everything you tried for your tinnitus prior to PTM. For each effort, what were you hoping would happen, and what actually did happen? *[Note: Sometimes a pattern will emerge showing that repeated (unsuccessful) attempts were made to make the tinnitus quieter, resulting in frustration and distress. If this is the case, try to see this pattern more clearly.]*

What have you tried for tinnitus prior to PTM?	What were you hoping would happen?	What actually did happen?
_____	_____	_____
_____	_____	_____
_____	_____	_____
_____	_____	_____
_____	_____	_____
_____	_____	_____

5. Please describe the sounds you have used to manage your reactions to tinnitus since starting PTM. For each sound you tried, what were you hoping would happen, and what actually did happen? *(If you have the Sound Plan Worksheets that were used during Level 3, these can be used as a guide. It's also important to reinforce the idea that with PTM the goal is not to change the tinnitus, but rather to change how one feels.)*

What sounds have you used to manage reactions to tinnitus during PTM?	What were you hoping would happen?	What actually did happen?

6. If you decide to move ahead with one-on-one support, then we will be making plans for using sound to manage your reactions to tinnitus. It will be helpful to have a list of sound-producing devices that you have available to you. Which of the following devices do you own? (For each type of device listed below, provide additional details. For instance, if you own a radio, how many radios do you have? Are any of them portable? If not portable, where are they located? For each device you own, how is it currently being used for tinnitus management?)

Type of device	How many are available?	Are any portable?	If not portable, where is it located?	How is it being used with respect to tinnitus?
☐ Television (smartTV? music channels available?)				
☐ Computer with internet (to access YouTube, radio stations, podcasts, etc.)				
☐ Smartphone capable of playing music and podcasts				
☐ Traditional radio				
☐ Satellite radio				
☐ CD or DVD player				
☐ Tabletop sound generator				
☐ Tabletop water fountain				
☐ Fan/air conditioner/etc.				
☐ Other				

About the Author

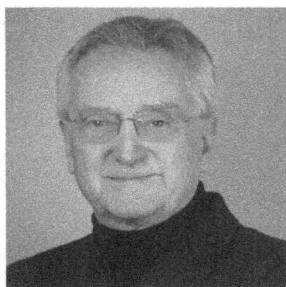

James A. Henry, PhD, is an audiologist with a doctorate in behavioral neuroscience. His six years earning his doctorate under the mentorship of Dr. Mary Meikle at the Oregon Hearing Research Center (OHRC—Dr. Jack Vernon was Director) ignited a passionate interest in conducting tinnitus research. During his professional career of over 35 years, he received funding of $28 million as principal or co-principal investigator for 43 projects and grants. He has authored over 250 publications, including more than 140 articles in peer-reviewed journals and seven books about tinnitus (this one is his eighth). He gave lectures and presentations nationally and internationally. His accomplishments resulted in numerous awards, including the Veterans Affairs (VA) Rehabilitation Research and Development 2016 Paul B. Magnuson Award *("the highest honor for VA rehabilitation investigators")* and the Jerger Career Award for Research in Audiology from the American Academy of Audiology Honors Committee.

Dr. Henry, who retired in 2022, continues to give lectures and training workshops, serves as an expert consultant, and has maintained his role as editor-at-large for the American Tinnitus Association's journal *Tinnitus Today*. His primary interest, however, is writing books about tinnitus, sound-hypersensitivity disorders, and hearing loss. This book is the third in a series of books he has planned under his corporation Ears Gone Wrong, LLC.

The target audience for these books is both healthcare professionals and the lay public. The books are written with the rigor that is required for peer-reviewed journals, including hundreds of references to support the text. To make the books more accessible, technical and medical terms are minimized, and explained when used. Writing in this manner makes the books accessible to professionals in all healthcare disciplines as well as the general public.

Dr. Henry's website is https://www.earsgonewrong.org/.

Acknowledgments

I hardly know where to start to properly acknowledge the many people who have contributed directly and indirectly to this book. I'll start by dedicating the book to Paula Myers, PhD, Carolyn Schmidt, PhD, and Tara Zaugg, AuD—the co-founders of PTM. I am indebted to each of these individuals for their enormous contributions to make PTM a reality. Together, we were the "fearsome foursome" who worked together for years to create PTM, conduct research trials, publish books and articles about PTM, develop online training programs, and present in-person training seminars.

Certain individuals made significant contributions to the development and refining of PTM, including Katie Edmonds, Marie-Christine Goodworth, Christine Kaelin, Idalisse Martinez, Cheryl Ribbe, and Emily Thielman. Many of these individuals continue to collaborate to improve different aspects of PTM and create materials and training to optimize its use in the clinic.

My 35-year career was supported primarily by the Veterans Affairs (VA) Rehabilitation Research & Development

(RR&D) Service. In essence, they kept me funded for that entire period of time to conduct and publish my research. I am indebted to RR&D, which also has funded the National Center for Rehabilitative Auditory Research (NCRAR) since 1997. I worked at the NCRAR from the time of its inception until I retired. I am indebted to Dr. Stephen Fausti, the Founder and Director of the NCRAR who was always supportive of my research. Dr. Fausti retired and was replaced by Dr. M. Patrick Feeney who was likewise very supportive.

Significant edits were made by my wife, Mary Jo who has a gift for making scientific language more accessible.

The book was proofread and copyedited by Robin L. Reed. Formatting of the book and book cover was done by Masha Shubin of Anno Domini Creative. Special thanks to both of them for their fine work.

References

1. Vernon JA, Schleuning A, Odell L, Hughes F. A tinnitus clinic. *Ear Nose and Throat Journal.* 1977;56:58–71.

2. Henry JA, Meikle MB. Pulsed versus continuous tones for evaluating the loudness of tinnitus. *Journal of the American Academy of Audiology.* 1999;10(5):261-72.

3. Henry JA. Loudness recruitment only partially explains the small size of tinnitus loudness-matches. In: Reich GE, Vernon JA, eds. *Proceedings of the Fifth International Tinnitus Seminar 1995.* American Tinnitus Association; 1996:148-157.

4. Henry JA. *The Tinnitus Book: Understanding Tinnitus and How To Find Relief.* Ears Gone Wrong, LLC. 2023.

5. Henry JA. *The Tinnitus Retraining Therapy Book: Walking You Through TRT.* Ears Gone Wrong, LLC; 2024.

6.	Davison GC. Stepped care: doing more with less? *Journal of Consulting and Clinical Psychology.* 2000;68(4):580-5.

7.	Henry JA, Griest S, Austin D, et al. Tinnitus Screener: Results from the first 100 participants in an epidemiology study. *American Journal of Audiology.* 2016;25(2):153-60. doi:10.1044/2016_AJA-15-0076

8.	Thielman EJ, Reavis KM, Theodoroff SM, et al. Tinnitus Screener: Short-term test-retest reliability. *American Journal of Audiology.* 2023;32(1):232-242. doi:10.1044/2022_AJA-22-00140

9.	Henry JA, Dennis KC, Schechter MA. General review of tinnitus: prevalence, mechanisms, effects, and management. *Journal of Speech Language and Hearing Research.* 2005;48(5):1204-35. doi:10.1044/1092-4388(2005/084)

10.	Axelsson A, Prasher D. Tinnitus induced by occupational and leisure noise. *Noise and Health.* 2000;2(8):47-54.

11.	Altissimi G, Colizza A, Cianfrone G, et al. Drugs inducing hearing loss, tinnitus, dizziness and vertigo: an updated guide. *European Review for Medical and Pharmacological Sciences.* 2020;24(15):7946-7952. doi:10.26355/eurrev_202008_22477

12.	DiSogra RM. Common aminoglycosides and platinum-based ototoxic drugs: Cochlear/vestibular side effects and incidence. *Seminars in Hearing.* 2019;40(2):104-107. doi:10.1055/s-0039-1684040

13. Dille MF, Konrad-Martin D, Gallun F, et al. Tinnitus onset rates from chemotherapeutic agents and ototoxic antibiotics: results of a large prospective study. *Journal of the American Academy of Audiology.* 2010;21(6):409-17. doi:10.3766/jaaa.21.6.6

14. Tunkel DE, Bauer CA, Sun GH, et al. Clinical practice guideline: tinnitus. *Otolaryngology Head and Neck Surgery.* 2014;151(2 Suppl):S1-S40. doi:10.1177/0194599814545325

15. 20Q: Tinnitus – options for clinical evaluation and treatment. AudiologyOnline, Article 28521.

16. Henry JA, McMillan L, Manning C. Multidisciplinary tinnitus care. *The Journal for Nurse Practitioners.* 2019;15:671-675.

17. Newman CW, Sandridge SA, Jacobson GP. Assessing outcomes of tinnitus intervention. *Journal of the American Academy of Audiology.* 2014;25(1):76-105. doi:10.3766/jaaa.25.1.6

18. Theodoroff SM. Tinnitus questionnaires for research and clinical use. *Current Topics in Behavioral Neuroscience.* 2021;51:403-418. doi:10.1007/7854_2020_175

19. Tyler RS. Tinnitus disability and handicap questionnaires. *Seminars in Hearing.* 1993;14:377-383.

20. Meikle MB, Henry JA, Griest SE, et al. The Tinnitus Functional Index: development of a new clinical measure for chronic, intrusive tinnitus. *Ear and Hearing.* 2012;33(2):153-76. doi:10.1097/AUD.0b013e31822f67c0

21. Hoffman HJ, Reed GW. Epidemiology of tinnitus. In: Snow JB, ed. *Tinnitus: Theory and Management.* BC Decker Inc.; 2004:16-41.

22. Jarach CM, Lugo A, Scala M, et al. Global prevalence and incidence of tinnitus: a systematic review and meta-analysis. *JAMA Neurology.* 2022;79(9):888-900. doi:10.1001/jamaneurol.2022.2189

23. Fagelson M. Tinnitus and traumatic memory. *Brain Science.* 2022;12(11)doi:10.3390/brainsci12111585

24. Kreuzer PM, Landgrebe M, Vielsmeier V, Kleinjung T, De Ridder D, Langguth B. Trauma-associated tinnitus. *Journal of Head Trauma Rehabilitation.* 2014;29(5):432-42. doi:10.1097/HTR.0b013e31829d3129

25. Fagelson MA. The association between tinnitus and posttraumatic stress disorder. *American Journal of Audiology.* 2007;16(2):107-17. doi:10.1044/1059-0889(2007/015)

26. Mazurek B, Boecking B, Brueggemann P. Association between stress and tinnitus-new aspects. *Otology and Neurotology.* 2019;40(4):e467-e473. doi:10.1097/ MAO.0000000000002180

27. Weise C, Hesser H, Andersson G, et al. The role of catastrophizing in recent onset tinnitus: its nature and association with tinnitus distress and medical utilization. *International Journal of Audiology.* 2013;52(3):177-88. doi:10.3109/14992027.2012.752111

28. Dobie RA. Overview: suffering from tinnitus. In: Snow JB, ed. *Tinnitus: Theory and Management.* BC Decker Inc; 2004:1-7.

29. House P. Personality of the tinnitus patient. In: Evered D, Lawrenson G, eds. *CIBA Foundation Symposium 85*. Pitman; 1981:193-198.

30. Langenbach M, Olderog M, Michel O, Albus C, Kohle K. Psychosocial and personality predictors of tinnitus-related distress. *General Hospital Psychiatry*. 2005;27(1):73-7. doi:10.1016/j.genhosppsych.2004.08.008

31. Reich GE, Johnson RM. Personality characteristics of tinnitus patients. *Journal of Laryngology and Otology (Suppl)*. 1984;9:228–232.

32. Unterrainer J, Greimel KV, Leibetseder M, Koller T. Experiencing tinnitus: which factors are important for perceived severity of the symptom? *International Tinnitus Journal*. 2003;9(2):130-3.

33. Durai M, Searchfield GD. A mixed-methods trial of broad band noise and nature sounds for tinnitus therapy: group and individual responses modeled under the adaptation level theory of tinnitus. *Frontiers in Aging Neuroscience*. 2017;9:44. doi:10.3389/fnagi.2017.00044

34. Hillecke T, Nickel A, Bolay HV. Scientific perspectives on music therapy. *Annals of the New York Academy of Science*. 2005;1060:271-82. doi:10.1196/annals.1360.020

35. Labbe E, Schmidt N, Babin J, Pharr M. Coping with stress: the effectiveness of different types of music. *Applied Psychophysiological Biofeedback*. 2007;32(3-4):163-8. doi:10.1007/s10484-007-9043-9

36. Felix M, Ferreira MBG, da Cruz LF, Barbosa MH. Relaxation therapy with guided imagery for post-operative pain management: An integrative review. *Pain Management Nursing.* 2019;20(1):3-9. doi:10.1016/j.pmn.2017.10.014

37. Skagerstrand A, Kobler S, Stenfelt S. Loudness and annoyance of disturbing sounds - perception by normal hearing subjects. *International Journal of Audiology.* 2017;56(10):775-783. doi:10.1080/14992027.2017.1321790

38. Zaman R, Hankir A, Jemni M. Lifestyle factors and mental health. *Psychiatria Danubia.* 2019;31(Suppl 3):217-220.

39. Jansen C, Le Prell C, Spankovich C. Health determinants and modifiable risk factors of tinnitus. In: Deshpande AK, Hall JWI, eds. *Tinnitus: Advances in Prevention, Assessment, and Management.* Plural Publishing; 2022:41-69.

40. Henry JA, Quinn CM. Sound therapy for tinnitus: options for audiologists. *Perspectives of the ASHA Special Interest Groups, SIG 8.* 2020;5:669-683.

41. Trevino M, Trehan A, Escabi CD, Lobarinas E. Mechanisms of noise- and music-induced tinnitus. In: Deshpande AK, Hall JWI, eds. *Tinnitus: Advances in Prevention, Assessment, and Management.* Plural Publishing; 2022:3-21.

42. Pienkowski M. Loud music and leisure noise is a common cause of chronic hearing loss, tinnitus and hyperacusis. *International Journal of Environmental Research and Public Health*. 2021;18(8)doi:10.3390/ ijerph18084236

43. Hahad O, Prochaska JH, Daiber A, Muenzel T. Environmental noise-induced effects on stress hormones, oxidative stress, and vascular dysfunction: key factors in the relationship between cerebrocardiovascular and psychological disorders. *Oxidative Medicine and Cellular Longevity*. 2019;2019:4623109. doi:10.1155/2019/4623109

44. Jastreboff PJ. Tinnitus. In: Gates GA, ed. *Current Therapy in Otolaryngology–Head and Neck Surgery*. 6 ed. Mosby-YearBook, Inc.; 1998:90–95.

45. Jastreboff PJ. Categories of the patients in TRT and the treatment outcome. In: Hazell JWP, ed. *Proceedings of the Sixth International Tinnitus Seminar 1999*. The Tinnitus and Hyperacusis Centre; 1999:394-398.

46. Jastreboff PJ. Tinnitus Retraining Therapy. In: Moller AR, Langguth B, DeRidder D, Kleinjung T, eds. *Textbook of Tinnitus*. Springer; 2011:575-596.

47. McFerran DJ, Stockdale D, Holme R, Large CH, Baguley DM. Why is there no cure for tinnitus? *Frontiers in Neuroscience*. 2019;13:802. doi:10.3389/ fnins.2019.00802

48. Vernon JA. Relief of tinnitus by masking treatment. In: English GM, ed. *Otolaryngology*. Harper & Row; 1982:1-21.

49. Jastreboff PJ, Hazell JWP. *Tinnitus Retraining Therapy: Implementing the Neurophysiological Model.* Cambridge University Press; 2004.

50. Henry JL, Wilson PH. *The Psychological Management of Chronic Tinnitus.* Allyn & Bacon; 2001.

51. Cima RF, Andersson G, Schmidt CJ, Henry JA. Cognitive-behavioral treatments for tinnitus: a review of the literature. *Journal of the American Academy of Audiology.* 2014;25(1):29-61. doi:10.3766/jaaa.25.1.4

52. Pantev C, Okamoto H, Teismann H. Music-induced cortical plasticity and lateral inhibition in the human auditory cortex as foundations for tonal tinnitus treatment. *Frontiers in Systems Neuroscience.* 2012;6:50. doi:10.3389/fnsys.2012.00050

53. Haab L, Lehser C, Corona-Strauss FI, et al. Implementation and long-term evaluation of a hearing aid supported tinnitus treatment using notched environmental sounds. *IEEE Journal of Translational Engineering in Health and Medicine.* 2019;7:1600109. doi:10.1109/JTEHM.2019.2897570

54. Marcrum SC, Picou EM, Steffens T, et al. Conventional versus notch filter amplification for the treatment of tinnitus in adults with mild-to-moderate hearing loss. *Progress in Brain Research.* 2021;260:235-252. doi:10.1016/bs.pbr.2020.06.020

55. Tziridis K, Brunner S, Schilling A, Krauss P, Schulze H. Spectrally matched near-threshold noise for subjective tinnitus loudness attenuation based on stochastic resonance. *Frontiers in Neuroscience.* 2022;16:831581. doi:10.3389/fnins.2022.831581

56. Schad ML, McMillan GP, Thielman EJ, et al. Comparison of acoustic therapies for tinnitus suppression: a preliminary trial. *International Journal of Audiology.* 2018;57(2):143-149. doi:10.1080/14992027.2017.1385862

57. Drexler D, Lopez-Paullier M, Rodio S, Gonzalez M, Geisinger D, Pedemonte M. Impact of reduction of tinnitus intensity on patients' quality of life. *International Journal of Audiology.* 2016;55(1):11-9. doi:10.3109/14992027.2015.1072772

58. Pedemonte M, Drexler D, Rodio S, et al. Tinnitus treatment with sound stimulation during sleep. *International Tinnitus Journal.* 2010;16(1):37-43.

59. Theodoroff SM, McMillan GP, Zaugg TL, Cheslock M, Roberts C, Henry JA. Randomized controlled trial of a novel device for tinnitus sound therapy during sleep. *American Journal of Audiology.* 2017;26(4):543-554. doi:10.1044/2017_AJA-17-0022

60. Henry JA, Thielman E, Zaugg T, et al. Development and field testing of a smartphone "App" for tinnitus management. *International Journal of Audiology.* 2017;56(10):784-792. doi:10.1080/14992027.2017.1338762

61. Kutyba JJ, Jedrzejczak WW, Gos E, Raj-Koziak D, Skarzynski PH. Chronic tinnitus and the positive effects of sound treatment via a smartphone app: mixed-design study. *JMIR Mhealth and Uhealth.* 2022;10(4):e33543. doi:10.2196/33543

62. Beukes EW, Andersson G, Manchaiah V, Kaldo V. *Cognitive Behavioral Therapy for Tinnitus.* Plural Publishing; 2021.

63. Beck JS. *Cognitive Therapy: Basics and Beyond.* Guilford; 1995.

64. Henry JA, Zaugg TL, Myers PJ, Kendall (Schmidt) CJ. *How to Manage Your Tinnitus: A Step-by-step Workbook, Third Edition.* Plural Publishing Inc.; 2010.

65. Schmidt CJ, Kaelin C, Henselman L, Henry JA. Need for mental health providers in Progressive Tinnitus Management: a gap in clinical care. *Federal Practitioner.* 2017;34(5):6-9.

66. Kahl KG, Winter L, Schweiger U. The third wave of cognitive behavioural therapies: what is new and what is effective? *Current Opinions in Psychiatry.* 2012;25(6):522-8. doi:10.1097/YCO.0b013e328358e531

67. Hayes SC, Hofmann SG. The third wave of Cognitive Behavioral Therapy and the rise of process-based care. *World Psychiatry.* 2017;16(3):245-246. doi:10.1002/wps.20442

68. Balandeh E, Omidi A, Ghaderi A. A narrative review of third-wave cognitive-behavioral therapies in addiction. *Addiction and Health.* 2021;13(1):52-65. doi:10.22122/ahj.v13i1.298

69. Apolinario-Hagen J, Druge M, Fritsche L. Cognitive behavioral therapy, mindfulness-based cognitive therapy and acceptance commitment therapy for anxiety disorders: Integrating traditional with dgital treatment approaches. *Advances in Experimental Medicine and Biology*. 2020;1191:291-329. doi:10.1007/978-981-32-9705-0_17

70. Westin VZ, Schulin M, Hesser H, et al. Acceptance and Commitment Therapy versus Tinnitus Retraining Therapy in the treatment of tinnitus: a randomised controlled trial. *Behaviour Research and Therapy*. 2011;49(11):737-47. doi:10.1016/j.brat.2011.08.001

71. Hesser H, Gustafsson T, Lunden C, et al. A randomized controlled trial of internet-delivered cognitive behavior therapy and acceptance and commitment therapy in the treatment of tinnitus. *Journal of Consulting and Clinical Psychology*. 2012;80(4):649-61. doi:10.1037/a0027021

72. Jastreboff PJ, Jastreboff MM. Tinnitus Retraining Therapy (TRT) as a method for treatment of tinnitus and hyperacusis patients. *Journal of the American Academy of Audiology*. 2000;11(3):162-77.

73. Mancini PC, Witt SA, Tyler RS, Perreau A. Establishing a tinnitus and hyperacusis clinic. In: Tyler RS, Perreau A, eds. *Tinnitus Treatment: Clinical Protocols*. 2 ed. Thieme; 2022:206-218.

74. Tyler RS, Haskell GB, Gogel SA, Gehringer AK. Establishing a tinnitus clinic in your practice. *American Journal of Audiology.* 2008;17(1):25-37. doi:10.1044/1059-0889(2008/004)

75. Perreau A, Tyler RS, Mancini PC, Witt SA. Tinnitus Activities Treatment. In: Tyler RS, Perreau A, eds. *Tinnitus Treatment: Clinical Protocols.* Thieme; 2022:42-70.

76. Tyler R, Ji H, Perreau A, Witt S, Noble W, Coelho C. Development and validation of the Tinnitus Primary Function Questionnaire. *American Journal of Audiology.* 2014;23(3):260-72. doi:10.1044/2014_AJA-13-0014

77. Tyler RS, Gehringer AK, Noble W, Dunn CC, Witt SA, Bardia A. Tinnitus Activities Treatment. In: Tyler RS, ed. *Tinnitus Treatment: Clinical protocols.* Thieme; 2006.

78. Tyler RS, Baker LJ. Difficulties experienced by tinnitus sufferers. *Journal of Speech and Hearing Disorders.* 1983;48(2):150–154. doi:10.1044/jshd.4802.150

79. Tyler RS, Gehringer AK, Noble W, Dunn CC, Witt SA, Bardia A. Tinnitus activities treatment. In: Tyler RS, ed. *Tinnitus Treatment: Clinical Protocols.* Thieme; 2006:116-132.

80. Henry JA, Sonstroem A, Smith B, Grush L. Survey of audiology graduate programs: training students in tinnitus management. *American Journal of Audiology.* 2021;30(1):22-27. doi:10.1044/2020_AJA-20-00140

81. Henry JA, Zaugg TL, Myers PM, Kendall CJ. *Progressive Tinnitus Management: Counseling Guide.* Plural Publishing; 2010.

82. Henry JA, Zaugg TL, Myers PM, Kendall (Schmidt) CJ. *Progressive Tinnitus Management: Clinical Handbook for Audiologists.* Plural Publishing; 2010.

83. Henry JA, Schechter MA, Loovis CL, Zaugg TL, Kaelin C, Montero M. Clinical management of tinnitus using a "progressive intervention" approach. *Journal of Rehabilitation Research and Development.* 2005;42(4 Suppl 2):95-116. doi:10.1682/jrrd.2005.01.0005

84. Husain FT, Gander PE, Jansen JN, Shen S. Expectations for tinnitus treatment and outcomes: A survey study of audiologists and patients. *Journal of the American Academy of Audiology.* 2018;29(4):313-336. doi:10.3766/jaaa.16154

85. Schmidt CJ, Kerns RD, Finkel S, Michaelides EM, Henry JA. Cognitive-behavioral therapy for Veterans with tinnitus. *Federal Practitioner.* 2018;35(8):36-46.

86. Henry JA, Goodworth MC, Lima E, Zaugg T, Thielman EJ. Cognitive Behavioral Therapy for tinnitus: Addressing the controversy of its clinical delivery by audiologists. *Ear and Hearing.* 2021;43(2):283-289. doi:10.1097/AUD.0000000000001150

87. Fuller TE, Haider HF, Kikidis D, et al. Different teams, same conclusions? A systematic review of existing clinical guidelines for the assessment and treatment of tinnitus in adults. *Frontiers in Psychology.* 2017;8:206. doi:10.3389/fpsyg.2017.00206

88. Cima RFF, Mazurek B, Haider H, et al. A multidisciplinary European guideline for tinnitus: diagnostics, assessment, and treatment. *HNO*. 2019;67(Suppl 1):10-42. doi:10.1007/s00106-019-0633-7

89. Langguth B, Kleinjung T, Schlee W, Vanneste S, De Ridder D. Tinnitus guidelines and their evidence base. *Journal of Clinical Medicine*. 2023;12(9) doi:10.3390/jcm12093087

90. Henry JA, Zaugg TL, Myers PJ, Kendall CJ, Michaelides EM. A triage guide for tinnitus. *Journal of Family Practice*. 2010;59(7):389-93.

91. Henry JA, Manning C. Clinical protocol to promote standardization of basic tinnitus services by audiologists. *American Journal of Audiology*. 2019;28(1S):152-161. doi:10.1044/2018_AJA-TTR17-18-0038

92. Henry JA. Sound therapy to reduce auditory gain for hyperacusis and tinnitus. *American Journal of Audiology*. 2022;31(4):1067-1077. doi:10.1044/2022_AJA-22-00127

93. Henry JA, Theodoroff SM, Edmonds C, et al. Sound tolerance conditions (hyperacusis, misophonia, noise sensitivity, and phonophobia): definitions and clinical management. *American Journal of Audiology*. 2022;31(3):513-527. doi:10.1044/2022_AJA-22-00035

94. Henry JA, Zaugg TL, Myers PJ, Kendall CJ, Turbin MB. Principles and application of educational counseling used in progressive audiologic tinnitus management. *Noise and Health*. 2009;11(42):33-48. doi:10.4103/1463-1741.45311

95. Henry JA, Thielman EJ, Zaugg TL, et al. Telephone-based Progressive Tinnitus Management for persons with and without traumatic brain injury: A randomized controlled trial. *Ear and Hearing*. 2019;40(2):227-242. doi:10.1097/AUD.0000000000000609

96. Henry JA, Thielman EJ, Zaugg TL, et al. Randomized controlled trial in clinical settings to evaluate effectiveness of coping skills education used with Progressive Tinnitus Management. *Journal of Speech Language and Hearing Research*. 2017;60(5):1378-1397. doi:10.1044/2016_JSLHR-H-16-0126

97. Henry JA, Zaugg TL, Myers PJ, Kendall (Schmidt) CJ. *How to Manage Your Tinnitus: A Step-by-step Workbook*. 3 ed. Plural Publishing Inc.; 2010.

98. Henry JA, Zaugg TL, Myers PJ, Kendall (Schmidt) CJ. *Progressive Tinnitus Management: Counseling Guide*. Plural Publishing Inc; 2010.

99. Andersson G. Psychological aspects of tinnitus and the application of cognitive-behavioral therapy. *Clinical Psychology Review*. 2002;22(7):977-90. doi:10.1016/s0272-7358(01)00124-6

100. Edmonds CM, Clark KD, Thielman EJ, Henry JA. Progressive Tinnitus Management Level 3 Skills Education: A 10-year clinical retrospective. *American Journal of Audiology.* 2022;31(3):567-578. doi:10.1044/2022_AJA-22-00003

101. Edmonds CM, Ribbe C, Thielman EJ, Henry JA. Progressive Tinnitus Management Level 3 Skills Education: A 5-year clinical retrospective. *American Journal of Audiology.* 2017;26(3):242-250. doi:10.1044/2017_AJA-16-0085

102. Langguth B, Biesinger E, Del Bo L, et al. Algorithm for the diagnostic and therapeutic management of tinnitus. In: Moller AR, Langguth B, DeRidder D, Kleinjung T, eds. *Textbook of Tinnitus.* Springer; 2011:381-385.

103. Newell S, Denneson L, Rynerson A, et al. Veterans Health Administration staff experiences with suicidal ideation screening and risk assessment in the context of COVID-19. *PLoS One.* 2021;16(12):e0261921. doi:10.1371/journal.pone.0261921

104. NIMH Brief Suicide Safety Assessment. National Institute of Mental Health (NIMH). Accessed September 19, 2023, https://www.nimh.nih.gov/research/research-conducted-at-nimh/asq-toolkit-materials/adult-outpatient/adult-outpatient-brief-suicide-safety-assessment-guide

105. Durai M, Searchfield G. Anxiety and depression, personality traits relevant to tinnitus: A scoping review. *International Journal of Audiology.* 2016;55(11):605-15. doi:10.1080/14992027.2016.1198966

106. Bartels H, Middel BL, van der Laan BF, Staal MJ, Albers FW. The additive effect of co-occurring anxiety and depression on health status, quality of life and coping strategies in help-seeking tinnitus sufferers. *Ear and Hearing.* 2008;29(6):947-56. doi:10.1097/AUD.0b013e3181888f83

107. Strumila R, Lengvenyte A, Vainutiene V, Lesinskas E. The role of questioning environment, personality traits, depressive and anxiety symptoms in tinnitus severity perception. *Psychiatry Quarterly.* 2017;88(4):865-877. doi:10.1007/s11126-017-9502-2

108. Salazar JW, Meisel K, Smith ER, Quiggle A, McCoy DB, Amans MR. Depression in patients with tinnitus: A systematic review. *Otolaryngology Head and Neck Surgery.* 2019;161(1):28-35. doi:10.1177/0194599819835178

109. Mencher GT, Gerber SE, McCombe A. *Audiology and Auditory Dysfunction.* Allyn & Bacon; 1997.

110. Schuknecht HF. *Pathology of the Ear.* 2 ed. Lea & Febiger; 1993.

111. Ridgway JM, Djalilian HR. Trauma to the ear. In: Djalilian HR, ed. *10 Minute ENT Consult.* Plural Publishing, Inc.; 2009:119-136.

112. Chandrasekhar SS, Tsai Do BS, Schwartz SR, et al. Clinical practice guideline: Sudden hearing loss (update). *Otolaryngology—Head and Neck Surgery*. 2019;161(1_suppl):S1-S45. doi:10.1177/0194599819859885

113. Fetterman BL, Saunders JE, Luxford WM. Prognosis and treatment of sudden sensorineural hearing loss. *Americal Journal of Otology*. 1996;17(4):529-36.

114. Goodhill V, Harris I. Sudden hearing loss syndrome. In: Goodhill V, ed. *Ear Diseases, Deafness and Dizziness*. Harper and Row; 1979.

115. Rothholtz VS, Djalilian HR. Hearing loss. In: Djalilian HR, ed. *10 Minute ENT Consult*. Plural Publishing, Inc.; 2009:75-93.

116. Jeyakumar A, Francis D, Doerr T. Treatment of idiopathic sudden sensorineural hearing loss. *Acta Otolaryngologica*. 2006;126(7):708-13. doi:10.1080/00016480500504234

117. Risbud A, Abouzari M, Djalilian HR. Case study 3: Pulsatile tinnitus. In: Deshpande AK, Hall JWI, eds. *Tinnitus: Advances in Prevention, Assessment, and Management*. Plural Publishing, Inc.; 2022:359-365.

118. Djalilian HR, Rothholtz VS, Hamidi S. Tinnitus. In: Djalilian HR, ed. *10 Minute ENT Consult*. Plural Publishing, Inc.; 2009:95-103.

119. Turner JJ. Otalgia and Otorrhea. In: Walker HK, Hall WD, Hurst JW, eds. *Clinical Methods: The History, Physical, and Laboratory Examinations*. 3rd ed. 1990.

120. Ely JW, Hansen MR, Clark EC. Diagnosis of ear pain. *American Family Physician*. 2008;77(5):621-8.

121. Danishyar A, Ashurst JV. Acute Otitis Media. *Stat-Pearls*. 2023.

122. Lee AD, Djalilian HR. Ear drainage. In: Djalilian HR, ed. *10 Minute ENT Consult*. Plural Publishing, Inc.; 2009:57-74.

123. Djalilian HR. Dizziness and vertigo. In: Djalilian HR, ed. *10 Minute ENT Consult*. Plural Publishing, Inc.; 2009:153-176.

124. Kim DK, Park SN, Kim HM, et al. Prevalence and significance of high-frequency hearing loss in subjectively normal-hearing patients with tinnitus. *Annals of Otology Rhinolology and Laryngology*. 2011;120(8):523-8. doi:10.1177/000348941112000806

125. Vernon JA, Meikle MB. Tinnitus masking. In: Tyler RS, ed. *Tinnitus Handbook*. Singular; 2000:313-356.

126. Henry JA, Reavis KM, Griest SE, et al. Tinnitus: an epidemiologic perspective. *Otolaryngology Clinics of North America*. 2020;53(4):481-499. doi:10.1016/j.otc.2020.03.002

127. Henry JA, Griest S, Zaugg TL, et al. Tinnitus and Hearing Survey: a screening tool to differentiate bothersome tinnitus from hearing difficulties. *American Journal of Audiology*. 2015;24(1):66-77. doi:10.1044/2014_AJA-14-0042

128. Kang HJ, Jin Z, Oh TI, et al. Audiologic characteristics of hearing and tinnitus in occupational noise-induced hearing loss. *The Journal of International Advanced Otology.* 2021;17(4):330-334. doi:10.5152/iao.2021.9259

129. Salvi R, Auerbach BD, Lau C, et al. Functional neuroanatomy of salicylate- and noise-induced tinnitus and hyperacusis. *Current Topics in Behavioral Neuroscience.* 2021;51:133-160. doi:10.1007/7854_2020_156

130. Spitzer RL, Kroenke K, Williams JB, Lowe B. A brief measure for assessing generalized anxiety disorder: the GAD-7. *Archives of Internal Medicine.* 2006;166(10):1092-7. doi:10.1001/archinte.166.10.1092

131. Rutter LA, Brown TA. Psychometric properties of the Generalized Anxiety Disorder Scale-7 (GAD-7) in outpatients with anxiety and mood disorders. *Journal of Psychopathological Behavioral Assessment.* 2017;39(1):140-146. doi:10.1007/s10862-016-9571-9

132. Plummer F, Manea L, Trepel D, McMillan D. Screening for anxiety disorders with the GAD-7 and GAD-2: a systematic review and diagnostic meta-analysis. *General Hospital Psychiatry.* 2016;39:24-31. doi:10.1016/j.genhosppsych.2015.11.005

133. Kroenke K, Spitzer RL, Williams JB. The PHQ-9: validity of a brief depression severity measure. *Journal of General Internal Medicine.* 2001;16(9):606-13. doi:10.1046/j.1525-1497.2001.016009606.x

134. Martin A, Rief W, Klaiberg A, Braehler E. Validity of the Brief Patient Health Questionnaire Mood Scale (PHQ-9) in the general population. *General Hospital Psychiatry*. 2006;28(1):71-7. doi:10.1016/j.genhosppsych.2005.07.003

135. Meikle M, Taylor-Walsh E. Characteristics of tinnitus and related observations in over 1800 tinnitus clinic patients. *Journal of Laryngology and Otology Supplement*. 1984;9:17-21. doi:10.1017/s1755146300090053

136. Erlandsson S. Psychological profiles of tinnitus patients. In: Tyler RS, ed. *Tinnitus Handbook*. Singular; 2000:25-57.

137. Bastien CH, Vallieres A, Morin CM. Validation of the Insomnia Severity Index as an outcome measure for insomnia research. *Sleep Medicine*. 2001;2(4):297-307. doi:10.1016/s1389-9457(00)00065-4

138. Lan T, Cao Z, Zhao F, Perham N. The association between effectiveness of tinnitus intervention and cognitive function-a systematic review. *Frontiers in Psychology*. 2020;11:553449. doi:10.3389/fpsyg.2020.553449

139. Clarke NA, Henshaw H, Akeroyd MA, Adams B, Hoare DJ. Associations between subjective tinnitus and cognitive performance: systematic review and meta-analyses. *Trends in Hearing*. 2020;24:2331216520918416. doi:10.1177/2331216520918416

140. Sherlock LP, Brungart DS. Functional impact of bothersome tinnitus on cognitive test performance. *International Journal of Audiology*. 2021;60(12):1000-1008. doi:10.1080/14992027.2021.1909760

141. Brueggemann P, Neff PKA, Meyer M, Riemer N, Rose M, Mazurek B. On the relationship between tinnitus distress, cognitive performance and aging. *Progress in Brain Research*. 2021;262:263-285. doi:10.1016/bs.pbr.2021.01.028

142. Nagaratnam JM, Sharmin S, Diker A, Lim WK, Maier AB. Trajectories of Mini-Mental State Examination scores over the lifespan in general populations: a systematic review and meta-regression analysis. *Clinical Gerontology*. 2022;45(3):467-476. doi:10.1080/07317115.2020.1756021

143. Andersson G, Marks E. Concentration. In: Tyler RS, ed. *The Consumer Handbook on Tinnitus*. 2 ed. Auricle Ink Publishers; 2016:163-178.

144. Henry JA, Schechter MA, Zaugg TL, et al. Clinical trial to compare tinnitus masking and tinnitus retraining therapy. *Acta Oto-Laryngologica Supplementum*. 2006;(556):64-9. doi:10.1080/03655230600895556

145. Ratnayake SA, Jayarajan V, Bartlett J. Could an underlying hearing loss be a significant factor in the handicap caused by tinnitus? *Noise and Health*. 2009;11(44):156-60. doi:10.4103/1463-1741.53362

146. Benson EA, Messersmith JJ. Audiologic assessment. *Seminars in Hearing*. 2022;43(2):58-65. doi:10.1055/s-0042-1749176

147. Sydlowski SA, King M, Petter K, Bachmann ML. Functional assessment of hearing aid benefit: Incorporating verification and aided speech recognition testing into routine practice. *Seminars in Hearing*. 2021;42(4):365-372. doi:10.1055/s-0041-1739369

148. Aristidou IL, Hohman MH. Central auditory processing disorder. *StatPearls*. 2023.

149. Evered D, Lawrenson G, eds. *Tinnitus. Ciba Foundation Symposium 85*. Pitman Books, Ltd.; 1981.

150. McFadden D. *Tinnitus—Facts, Theories and Treatments*. National Academy Press; 1982.

151. Henry JA, Meikle MB. Psychoacoustic measures of tinnitus. *Journal of the American Academy of Audiology*. 2000;11:138-155.

152. Henry JA. "Measurement" of tinnitus. *Otology and Neurotology*. 2016;37(8):e276-85. doi:10.1097/MAO.0000000000001070

153. Andersson G. Tinnitus loudness matchings in relation to annoyance and grading of severity. *Auris Nasus Larynx*. 2003;30(2):129-33. doi:10.1016/s0385-8146(03)00008-7

154. Colagrosso EMG, Fournier P, Fitzpatrick EM, Hebert S. A qualitative study on factors modulating tinnitus experience. *Ear and Hearing*. 2019;40(3):636-644. doi:10.1097/AUD.0000000000000642

155. Vidal JL, Park JM, Han JS, Alshaikh H, Park SN. Measurement of loudness discomfort levels as a test for hyperacusis: test-retest reliability and its clinical value. *Clinical and Experimental Otorhinolaryngology*. 2022;15(1):84-90. doi:10.21053/ceo.2021.00318

156. Henry JA. Distinguishing between hearing loss, tinnitus, and hyperacusis: A recommended tinnitus-evaluation protocol for audiologists. *Tinnitus Today*. 2020;45(1):22-27.

157. Zaugg TL, Thielman EJ, Griest S, Henry JA. Subjective reports of trouble tolerating sound in daily life versus loudness discomfort levels. *American Journal of Audiology*. 2016;25(4):359-363. doi:10.1044/2016_AJA-15-0034

158. Henry JA. Considering Tinnitus Management Versus Cure. *Tinnitus Today*. 2021;46(1):10-11.

159. Henry JA, Thielman EJ, Zaugg T, Griest S, Stewart BJ. Assessing meaningful improvement: focus on the Tinnitus Functional Index. *Ear and Hearing*. 2024;doi:10.1097/AUD.0000000000001456

160. Schechter MA, Henry JA. Assessment and treatment of tinnitus patients using a "masking approach". *Journal of the American Academy of Audiology*. 2002;13(10):545-58.

161. Martinez Devesa P, Waddell A, Perera R, Theodoulou M. Cognitive behavioural therapy for tinnitus. *Cochrane Database Systematic Review*. 2007;(1):CD005233. doi:10.1002/14651858.CD005233.pub2

162. Schmidt CJ, Kerns RD, Finkel S, Michaelides E, Henry JA. Cognitive behavioral therapy for Veterans with tinnitus. *Federal Practitioner.* 2018;35(8):36-46.

163. Henry JA, Rheinsburg B, Zaugg T. Comparison of custom sounds for achieving tinnitus relief. *Journal of the American Academy of Audiology.* 2004;15(8):585-98. doi:10.3766/jaaa.15.8.6

164. Johnson MH. How does distraction work in the management of pain? *Current Pain and Headache Reports.* 2005;9(2):90-5. doi:10.1007/s11916-005-0044-1

165. Bascour-Sandoval C, Salgado-Salgado S, Gomez-Milan E, Fernandez-Gomez J, Michael GA, Galvez-Garcia G. Pain and distraction according to sensory modalities: current findings and future directions. *Pain Practice.* 2019;19(7):686-702. doi:10.1111/papr.12799

166. Henry JA. If you don't listen to it, it's not really a problem. *Tinnitus Today.* 2004;29:16-17.

167. Henry JA. Directed attention and habituation: two concepts critical to tinnitus management. *American Journal of Audiology.* 2023:1-8. doi:10.1044/2022_AJA-22-00178

168. Henry JA, Trune DR, Robb MJA, Jastreboff PJ. *Tinnitus Retraining Therapy: Clinical Guidelines.* Plural Publishing, Inc.; 2007.

169. Henry JA, Zaugg T, Schechter MA. Clinical guide for audiologic tinnitus management I: Assessment. *Am J Audiol.* 2005;14:21-48.

170. Martinez-Devesa P, Perera R, Theodoulou M, Waddell A. Cognitive behavioural therapy for tinnitus. *Cochrane Database Systematic Review.* 2010;(9):CD005233. doi:10.1002/14651858.CD005233.pub3

171. Bandura A. Health promotion by social cognitive means. *Health Education & Behavior.* 2004;31(2):143-64. doi:10.1177/1090198104263660

172. Sweetow RW. Cognitive aspects of tinnitus patient management. *Ear and Hearing.* 1986;7(6):390-6. doi:10.1097/00003446-198612000-00008

173. Sweetow RW. Counseling the patient with tinnitus. *Archives of Otolaryngology.* 1985;111(5):283-4.

174. Andersson G, Kaldo V. Cognitive-Behavioral Therapy with applied relaxation. In: Tyler RS, ed. *Tinnitus Treatment: Clinical Protocols.* Thieme Medical Publishers, Inc.; 2006:96-115.

175. Fuller T, Cima R, Langguth B, Mazurek B, Vlaeyen JW, Hoare DJ. Cognitive Behavioural Therapy for tinnitus. *Cochrane Database Systematic Review.* 2020;1(1):CD012614. doi:10.1002/14651858.CD012614.pub2

176. Beukes EW, Baguley DM, Allen PM, Manchaiah V, Andersson G. Audiologist-guided internet-based cognitive behavior therapy for adults with tinnitus in the United Kingdom: a randomized controlled trial. *Ear and Hearing.* 2018;39(3):423-433. doi:10.1097/AUD.0000000000000505

177. Weise C, Kleinstauber M, Andersson G. Internet-delivered cognitive-behavior therapy for tinnitus: a randomized controlled trial. *Psychosomatic Medicine*. 2016;78(4):501-10. doi:10.1097/PSY.0000000000000310

178. Henry JA, Goodworth MC, Lima E, Zaugg T, Thielman EJ. Cognitive Behavioral Therapy for tinnitus: Addressing the controversy of its clinical delivery by audiologists. *Ear and Hearing*. 2022;43(2):283-289. doi:10.1097/AUD.0000000000001150

179. Henry JA, Zaugg TL, Schechter MA. Clinical guide for audiologic tinnitus management II: Treatment. *American Journal of Audiology*. 2005;14(1):49-70. doi:10.1044/1059-0889(2005/005)

180. Henry JL, Wilson PH. *Tinnitus: A Self-Management Guide for the Ringing in Your Ears*. Allyn & Bacon; 2002.

181. Formby C, Gold SL. Modification of loudness discomfort level: evidence for adaptive chronic auditory gain and its clinical relevance. *Seminars in Hearing*. 2002;23:21-35.

182. Iankilevitch M, Singh G, Russo FA. A scoping review and field guide of theoretical approaches and recommendations to studying the decision to adopt hearing aids. *Ear and Hearing*. 2023;44(3):460-476. doi:10.1097/AUD.0000000000001311

183. Kam ACS. Efficacy of amplification for tinnitus relief in people with mild hearing loss. *Journal of Speech Language and Hearing Research*. 2024;67(2):606-617. doi:10.1044/2023_JSLHR-23-00031

184. Jacquemin L, Gilles A, Shekhawat GS. Hearing more to hear less: a scoping review of hearing aids for tinnitus relief. *International Journal of Audiology*. 2022;61(11):887-895. doi:10.1080/14992027.2021.2007423

185. Shekhawat GS, Searchfield GD, Stinear CM. Role of hearing AIDS in tinnitus intervention: a scoping review. *Journal of the American Academy of Audiology*. 2013;24(8):747-62. doi:10.3766/jaaa.24.8.11

186. Henry JA, Frederick M, Sell S, Griest S, Abrams H. Validation of a novel combination hearing aid and tinnitus therapy device. *Ear and Hearing*. 2015;36(1):42-52. doi:10.1097/AUD.0000000000000093

187. Henry JA, McMillan G, Dann S, et al. Tinnitus management: randomized controlled trial comparing extended-wear hearing aids, conventional hearing aids, and combination instruments. *Journal of the American Academy of Audiology*. 2017;28(6):546-561. doi:10.3766/jaaa.16067

188. Waechter S, Olovsson M, Pettersson P. Should tinnitus patients with subclinical hearing impairment be offered hearing aids? A comparison of tinnitus mitigation following 3 months hearing aid use in individuals with and without clinical hearing impairment. *Journal of Clinical Medicine*. 2023;12(24) doi:10.3390/jcm12247660

189. Mealings K, Valderrama JT, Mejia J, Yeend I, Beach EF, Edwards B. Hearing aids reduce self-perceived difficulties in noise for listeners with normal audiograms. *Ear and Hearing.* 2024;45(1):151-163. doi:10.1097/AUD.0000000000001412

190. Mealings K, Yeend I, Valderrama JT, et al. Discovering the unmet needs of people with difficulties understanding speech in noise and a normal or near-normal audiogram. *American Journal of Audiology.* 2020;29(3):329-355. doi:10.1044/2020_AJA-19-00093

191. Hallam RS, Jakes SC, Hinchcliffe R. Cognitive variables in tinnitus annoyance. *British Journal of Clinical Psychology.* 1988;27(3):213-22. doi:10.1111/j.2044-8260.1988.tb00778.x

192. Andersson G, Baguley DM, McKenna L, McFerran D. *Tinnitus: A Multidisciplinary Approach.* Whurr Publishers Ltd; 2005.

193. McKenna L, Daniel HC. Tinnitus-related insomnia treatment. In: Tyler RS, ed. *Tinnitus Treatment: Clinical Protocols.* Thieme; 2006:81-95.

194. McKenna L, Marks E. The psychological management of tinnitus-related insomnia. In: Tyler RS, Perreau A, eds. *Tinnitus Treatment: Clinical Protocols.* Thieme; 2022:82-95.

195. Johns MW. A new method for measuring daytime sleepiness: the Epworth sleepiness scale. *Sleep.* 1991;14(6):540-5. doi:10.1093/sleep/14.6.540

196. Goncalves MT, Malafaia S, Moutinho Dos Santos J, Roth T, Marques DR. Epworth sleepiness scale: A meta-analytic study on the internal consistency. *Sleep Medicine*. 2023;109:261-269. doi:10.1016/j.sleep.2023.07.008

197. Buysse DJ, Reynolds CF, 3rd, Monk TH, Berman SR, Kupfer DJ. The Pittsburgh Sleep Quality Index: a new instrument for psychiatric practice and research. *Psychiatry Research*. 1989;28(2):193-213. doi:10.1016/0165-1781(89)90047-4

198. Lin J, Suurna M. Sleep apnea and sleep-disordered breathing. *Otolaryngologic Clinics of North America*. 2018;51(4):827-833. doi:10.1016/j.otc.2018.03.009

199. Howell M, Avidan AY, Foldvary-Schaefer N, et al. Management of REM sleep behavior disorder: an American Academy of Sleep Medicine clinical practice guideline. *J Clin Sleep Med*. Apr 1 2023;19(4):759-768. doi:10.5664/jcsm.10424

200. McCarter SJ, Howell MJ. Importance of rapid eye movement sleep behavior disorder to the primary care physician. *Mayo Clinic Proceedings*. 2016;91(10):1460-1466. doi:10.1016/j.mayocp.2016.07.019

201. Mehra R. Sleep apnea and the heart. *Cleveland Clinic Journal of Medicine*. 2019;86(9 Suppl 1):10-18. doi:10.3949/ccjm.86.s1.03

202. Bhatt JM, Bhattacharyya N, Lin HW. Relationships between tinnitus and the prevalence of anxiety and depression. *Laryngoscope*. 2017;127(2):466-469. doi:10.1002/lary.26107

203. Zigmond AS, Snaith RP. The hospital anxiety and depression scale. *Acta Psychiatrica Scandinavica.* 1983;67(6):361-70. doi:10.1111/j.1600-0447.1983. tb09716.x

204. Julian LJ. Measures of anxiety: State-Trait Anxiety Inventory (STAI), Beck Anxiety Inventory (BAI), and Hospital Anxiety and Depression Scale-Anxiety (HADS-A). *Arthritis Care Research (Hoboken).* 2011;63 Suppl 11(0 11):S467-72. doi:10.1002/acr.20561

205. Smarr KL, Keefer AL. Measures of depression and depressive symptoms: Beck Depression Inventory-II (BDI-II), Center for Epidemiologic Studies Depression Scale (CES-D), Geriatric Depression Scale (GDS), Hospital Anxiety and Depression Scale (HADS), and Patient Health Questionnaire-9 (PHQ-9). *Arthritis Care Research (Hoboken).* 2011;63 Suppl 11:S454-66. doi:10.1002/acr.20556

206. Sindhusake D, Golding M, Wigney D, Newall P, Jakobsen K, Mitchell P. Factors predicting severity of tinnitus: a population-based assessment. *Journal of the American Academy of Audiology.* 2004;15(4):269-80. doi:10.3766/jaaa.15.4.2

207. Folmer RL, Griest SE. Chronic tinnitus resulting from head or neck injuries. *Laryngoscope.* 2003;113(5):821-7. doi:10.1097/00005537-200305000-00010

208. Henry JA, Zaugg TL, Myers PJ, et al. Pilot study to develop telehealth tinnitus management for persons with and without traumatic brain injury. *Journal of Rehabilitation Research and Development.* 2012;49(7):1025-42. doi:10.1682/jrrd.2010.07.0125

209. Eilert N, Timulak L, Duffy D, et al. Following up internet-delivered cognitive behaviour therapy (CBT): A longitudinal qualitative investigation of clients' usage of CBT skills. *Clinical Psychology and Psychotherapy.* 2022;29(1):200-221. doi:10.1002/cpp.2619

210. Andersson G. Internet-delivered psychological treatments for tinnitus: A brief historical review. *American Journal of Audiology.* 2022;31(3S):1013-1018. doi:10.1044/2022_AJA-21-00245

211. Tyler RS, Perreau A, eds. *Tinnitus Treatment: Clinical Protocols.* 2 ed. Thieme; 2022.

212. Deshpande AK, Hall JWI, eds. *Tinnitus: Advances in Prevention, Assessment, and Management.* Plural Publishing; 2022.

213. Snow JB, ed. *Tinnitus: Theory and Management.* BC Decker Inc; 2004.

214. Moller AR, Langguth B, DeRidder D, Kleinjung T, eds. *Textbook of Tinnitus.* Springer; 2011.

215. Tyler RS, ed. *The Consumer Handbook on Tinnitus.* 2nd ed. Auricle Ink Publishers; 2016.

216. DiSogra RM, O'Brien-Russo CA, Deshpande AK. Dietary supplements, essential oils, and cannabinoids for tinnitus relief. In: Deshpande AK, Hall JWI, eds. *Tinnitus: Advances in Prevention, Assessment, and Management*. Plural Publishing; 2022:247-260.

217. Sackett DL. The fall of "clinical research" and the rise of "clinical-practice research". *Clinical Investigational Medicine*. 2000;23(6):379-81.

218. Henry JA, Thielman EJ, Grush LD. Application of teleudiology to the clinical management of tinnitus. In: Deshpande AK, Hall JWI, eds. *Tinnitus: Advances in Prevention, Assessment, and Management*. Plural Publishing; 2023:209-219.

219. Hoare DJ, Edmondson-Jones M, Sereda M, Akeroyd MA, Hall D. Amplification with hearing aids for patients with tinnitus and co-existing hearing loss. *Cochrane Database Systematic Review*. 2014;(1):CD010151. doi:10.1002/14651858.CD010151.pub2

220. McNeill C, Tavora-Vieira D, Alnafjan F, Searchfield GD, Welch D. Tinnitus pitch, masking, and the effectiveness of hearing aids for tinnitus therapy. *International Journal of Audiology*. 2012;51(12):914-9. doi:10.3109/14992027.2012.721934

221. Trotter MI, Donaldson I. Hearing aids and tinnitus therapy: a 25-year experience. *Journal of Laryngology and Otology*. 2008;122(10):1052-6. doi:10.1017/S002221510800203X

222. Beck JE, Zaugg TL, Egge JL, Lima EN, Thielman EJ. Progressive Tinnitus Management at two Veterans Affairs medical centers: Clinical implementation with modified protocols. *American Journal of Audiology.* 2019;28(1S):162-173. doi:10.1044/2018_AJA-TTR17-18-0040

223. Henry JA, Loovis C, Montero M, et al. Randomized clinical trial: group counseling based on tinnitus retraining therapy. *Journal of Rehabilitation Research and Development.* 2007;44(1):21-32. doi:10.1682/jrrd.2006.02.0018

224. Henry JA, Zaugg TL, Myers PJ, Schechter MA. Using therapeutic sound with progressive audiologic tinnitus management. *Trends in Amplification.* 2008;12(3):188-209. doi:10.1177/1084713808321184

225. Myers PJ, Griest S, Kaelin C, et al. Development of a progressive audiologic tinnitus management program for Veterans with tinnitus. *Journal of Rehabilitation Research and Development.* 2014;51(4):609-22. doi:10.1682/JRRD.2013.08.0189

226. Sherlock LP, Ortiz CE, Blasco GP, Brooks DI. Retrospective assessment of the efficacy of modified Progressive Tinnitus Management skills education in a military medical treatment facility. *Military Medicine.* 2019;184(9-10):e468-e473. doi:10.1093/milmed/usz024

227. Tuepker A, Elnitsky C, Newell S, Zaugg T, Henry JA. A qualitative study of implementation and adaptations to Progressive Tinnitus Management (PTM) delivery. *PLoS One*. 2018;13(5):e0196105. doi:10.1371/journal. pone.0196105

228. Zaugg TL, Thielman EJ, Carlson KF, et al. Factors affecting the implementation of evidence-based Progressive Tinnitus Management in Department of Veterans Affairs Medical Centers. *PLoS One*. 2020;15(12):e0242007. doi:10.1371/journal. pone.0242007

229. Henry JA, Folmer RL, Zaugg TL, et al. History of tinnitus research at the VA National Center for Rehabilitative Auditory Research (NCRAR), 1997-2021: Studies and key findings. *Seminars in Hearing*. 2023:1-25.

Index

www.ingramcontent.com/pod-product-compliance
Lightning Source LLC
Chambersburg PA
CBHW032050020426
42335CB00011B/277